The Everything Adrenal Fatigue Book

The Syndrome of Feeling Stressed-Out!

By: James M. Lowrance © 2010

TABLE OF CONTENTS:

SECTION ONE – (Pages 7 – 50):
"A Complete Look at Adrenal Fatigue"

CHAPTERS:

1. The Common Stress Syndrome
2. Medical Research Confirms the Existence of Mild Adrenal Insufficiency
3. More Detailed Symptoms of Adrenal Fatigue
4. Getting Tested for Adrenal Fatigue
5. My Personal Struggle with Adrenal Fatigue
6. Treatment for Adrenal Fatigue

TABLE OF CONTENTS:

SECTION TWO – (Pages 50 – 119): "The Best Darn CFS, Fibromyalgia and Adrenal Fatigue Book!"

CHAPTERS:

Common Symptoms of Chronic Fatigue Syndrome
2. The Suspected Causes of CFS
3. More on Dysautonomia in Chronic Fatigue Syndrome
4. Common Symptoms and Diagnosis of Fibromyalgia
5. Common Causes of Adrenal Fatigue Syndrome
6. Adrenal Fatigue or Adrenal Insufficiency?
7. The Accuracy of Saliva Adrenal Cortisol Testing
8. Cortisol Supplementation for Adrenal Fatigue
9. Boosting Fatigued Adrenal Glands
10. Diagnosing and Treating Addison's Disease (Autoimmune Adrenalitis)
11. How to Set Reasonable Health Goals
12. When is DHEA Supplementation Beneficial?

TABLE OF CONTENTS:

SECTION THREE – (Pages 120- 177): "Natural and Prescribed Treatments for Adrenal Fatigue"

CHAPTERS:

1. Adrenal Fatigue by Any Other Name
2. Adrenal Fatigue and Thyroid Patients
3. Balancing Adrenal Fatigue Treatment with Hypothyroid Therapy
4. Adrenal Fatigue or "Hypocortisolemia"
5. CFS, Fibromyalgia and Low Cortisol
6. Conditions That Cause Mild Adrenal Insufficiency
7. Cortisol & DHEA Supplements for Adrenal Fatigue
8. The Role Stress in Diseases and Syndromes
9. Another Look at Adrenal Fatigue Treatments
10. The Importance in Confirming Treatment Information

INTRODUCTION:

This comprehensive and complete e-book resource, covering symptoms, diagnosis and treatments for Adrenal Fatigue, contains 28 chapters. It is a compilation of three e-book titles authored by veteran health writer and Adrenal Fatigue patient- Jim Lowrance.

One important aspect covered within the chapters, is the fact that "cortisol supplementation" can be extremely valuable under the proper conditions and when administered by a qualified physician. If the treatment is not properly administered, "adrenal suppression" can result and other possible severe side-effects. There is not an anti-cortisol message in this e-book -- it is simply pointed-out that steroid cortisol treatment must be properly overseen and monitored when it becomes necessary. Natural methods for raising low cortisol levels in the body are suggested as a first-line trial to correct Adrenal Fatigue but the benefits of steroid cortisol are also given consideration within the chapters, for those who are found to be in need it (i.e. for severe adrenal exhaustion and Addison's disease).

It was the author's intention, to provide a complete source of information in easy-to-understand terms, so that both the novice reader and medical professional can benefit from the information contained in this e-book. Those who suffer Adrenal Fatigue conditions can find help and possible full recovery through the information provided in the chapters.

SECTION ONE – (Pages 7 – 50):
"A Complete Look at Adrenal Fatigue"

CHAPTER 1:

The Common Stress Syndrome

Adrenal fatigue is a common syndrome caused by chronic stress and affects a large percent of the population at some point in their lives (estimates are up to 80% of Americans), but if it can be recognized, it can also be treated.

While adrenal fatigue is not as serious as actual adrenal diseases and full-blown adrenal insufficiency, the symptoms can still be concerning and can also negatively affect a person's quality of life. With Adrenal Fatigue, as with more severe adrenal insufficient states, the hormone "Cortisol" is most commonly the one that becomes low or deficient. It is the hormone that manages stress in the body on a daily basis and provides energy for the body, in a cyclic rhythm.

A number of research articles going back more than 15 years, recognize mild adrenal dysfunction or a sub-clinically low functioning of the adrenal glands. This includes research articles on Chronic Fatigue Syndrome (CFS), Fibromyalgia and Post Traumatic Stress Disorder (PTSD), which have been proven in a number of medical research studies, to present with low cortisol levels. This condition, which causes characteristic symptoms (syndrome), has become increasingly common over the past several decades.

The main symptoms caused by Adrenal Fatigue, include the following.

• fatigue
• low tolerance for stress
• joint aches
• low tolerance for exercise
• irritability
• anxiety and depression
• low resistance to allergies and sicknesses
• sugar & salt cravings and over consumption of caffeine

The reason for the craving of these substances last mentioned is due to the need to supply energy from other sources, due to the person's adrenal glands having the diminished ability to do so.

This brings us to the understanding of what this syndrome actually is. It is a syndrome of the adrenals that have become exhausted, due to prolonged, chronic stress that has been placed upon them. The adrenal glands, which are two small glands, one sitting on each of our two kidneys, are designed to give the human body, the ability to handle and spring back from stress. They do this by means of releasing hormones that circulate throughout the body, giving it coping abilities and energies to deal with stressors. Stressors can be anything, mental or physical that put a demand of any kind on our bodies. This means stressors can be positive or negative but either type will place demands upon the adrenal glands.

The most important hormone released by the adrenals that help us deal with stress, is the one called "cortisol" or "cortical".

It, like the hormone adrenaline, is also a "fight or flight" hormone, the difference being that while adrenaline is the hormone to help us with immediate need for increased bodily functions to deal with tasks at hand needing performed, cortical, is the long-term fight or flight hormone, that gives us a steady ability to handle all of our everyday stressors.

CHAPTER 2:

Medical Research Confirms the Existence of Mild Adrenal Insufficiency

Stress is a known trigger for adrenal fatigue and related syndromes, such as Chronic Fatigue Syndrome and Fibromyalgia and it can also bring an autoimmune disease to the surface, that is in the body but hasn't fully manifested and thyroid diseases are some of the more common ones that are triggered by stress, especially Grave's Disease/hyperthyroidism. PTSD (Post Traumatic stress Disorder) is also a chronic stress caused syndrome but is also classified as an anxiety disorder.

Adrenal fatigue and the other syndromes that have adrenal fatigue as a feature have as one proposed cause, a blunted HPA Axis. This is referring to the group of endocrine glands that supply our bodies with needed hormone.

These glands are the Hypothalamus, Pituitary and Adrenals and they work in sync (axis) with each other but in these adrenal fatigue disorders, the response by these glands becomes "blunted" or slowed down, according to research that has been conducted.

A blunted HPA Axis is found commonly in conditions like CFS and Fibromyalgia and though some in the medical community believe this to be a bogus theory, there are many U.S. Gov/NIH medical studies to back it up. Because of this fact, adrenal fatigue syndromes should be looked at as real illnesses, with reputable medical research behind them. Many medical doctors do not seem to be aware of these findings as mentioned above but it is referred to by several departments of the National Institutes of Health, including the CDC, NIAMS and also The American Journal of Psychiatry.

What I like to point out about the medical research articles I cite in my own articles on the Adrenal Fatigue subject, is how clearly they recognize mild types of low adrenal function.

The one I Cite below is found from the PubMed (National Institutes of Health/National Library of Medicine) website and is among many that recognize Adrenal Fatigue type syndromes.

In the following research article link from PubMed the fact is cited that "early life stress" (ELS), can cause later-life low cortisol levels or what they term "hypocortisolemia".
(Research Link>
http://www.ncbi.nlm.nih.gov/pubmed/16399913)

The article is among many others that conclude that "stress" can be the cause of hypo-cortisolemia, cortisol being the adrenal hormone that moderates stress in the body but becomes inadequate with Adrenal Fatigue and Adrenal Insufficiency. This is why I refer to Adrenal Fatigue as a "stress syndrome". Ongoing stress (chronic) can have the very same effect in taxing the adrenals as do sudden traumatic experiences (Post Traumatic Stress). Despite the obvious, there are still some in the medical community who deny the existence of Adrenal Fatigue. Are they overlooking a significant number of medical research conclusions? Apparently they are.

For many years, sources that address the Adrenal Fatigue subject (though usually referred to by other names), point out that chronic stress first elevates cortisol but prolonged demand for this cortisol output, eventually exhausts/fatigues the adrenals and cortisol levels begin to deplete. Even medical research groups are missing this point that there is first high cortisol and afterward, it becomes chronically low with chronic or traumatic stress.

Following below, is another interesting PubMed article that points this fact out clearly and yet some researchers believe there is a contradiction when it actually confirms this very point in regard to cortisol first remaining chronically high and eventually falling to suppressed levels.

This research and the link, also from the PubMed website (National Institutes of Health) states that distressing events will first elevate cortisol levels but that long-term exposure to stress eventually disrupts the HPA Axis and results in cortisol levels dropping to sub-clinically low levels: (Research Link> http://www.ncbi.nlm.nih.gov/pubmed/11068377? dopt=Abstract)

The Everything Adrenal Fatigue Book

The preceding referenced research article gives a perfect description of what happens with Adrenal Fatigue syndromes and yet some in the medical community seem to be overlooking the obvious.

I suppose that the best thing for the time being is for the Adrenal Fatigue underground to continue informing the public until there is more widespread acknowledgment of this very real illness, that affects millions of people.

What really convinced me years ago, that mild adrenal dysfunction does exist and it has been proven in medical research, are those articles published in regard to syndromes like CFS, Fibromyalgia and PTSD (Post Traumatic Stress disorder). These articles clearly state that people with these type syndromes commonly suffer low cortisol levels and they have also found strong association of these syndromes to chronic stress, either prolonged or induced by sudden events.

Following are more example research articles and links:

This next link is to research published in 1996 by the National Institutes of health, stating that NIH researcher Dr. Straus and his colleagues found low cortisol levels in patients with CFS. They also state the fact that it has been long known that even subtle cortisol deficiency can cause lethargy and fatigue.
(Research Link>
http://www3.niaid.nih.gov/news/newsreleases/1998/cfs.htm)

In this next research article, also published by PubMed/NIH, it was concluded that both CFS and Fibromyalgia are "stress-response related" and abnormalities have been found in the "HPA Axis", the system of endocrine glands that regulate adrenal cortisol production. The study sites the fact that low cortisol has been found in patients with these stress related disorders, in contrast to high cortisol levels found in patients with depression.

They also mention the fact that single readings of cortisol may not be sufficient in determining low cortisol levels in these patients.
(Research Link>
http://www.pubmedcentral.nih.gov/articlerender.f cgi?artid=416440)

Some of the other things Medical Researchers have studied in regard to CFS and Fibromyalgia, is the fact that these syndromes can have different triggers for different patients but with many, it is an underlying viral, autoimmune, bacterial etc…, type infection in the body, that causes chronic activation of the immune system and over time, this uses up some of the adrenal reserves. The adrenals serve a major role in releasing cortisol, the body's natural anti-inflammatory, attempting to ward off inflammation.

Cortisol (also called "cortical"), is also the "stress hormone", that helps the body to deal with stresses of all kinds as previously mentioned, without it, even the smallest stressor would cause shock and death (adrenal crises).

It, along with adrenaline, are "fight or flight" hormones and help protect the body from the effects of stress, from minor emotional stress, to major ones, such as a car accident or serious disease.

This next research article link is from the publishers of the New England Journal of Medicine and states the fact that low cortisol production is often associated with people suffering from Post Traumatic Stress Disorder. (Research Link> http://psychiatry.jwatch.org/cgi/content/full/2007/1210/1)

While, research articles do not use the term "adrenal fatigue", this is exactly what is being described by them. They will instead use terms such as "mild adrenal insufficiency", "Blunted HPA axis", "hypocortisolism" and simply "low cortisol".

These type research articles are published in
significant numbers, so doctors who still do not
believe that sub-clinical adrenal insufficiency
exists, need to take a look at a few of these for
valid confirmation of this very real syndrome.

Adrenal fatigue by whatever other name they
wish to call by does exist and is found in a variety
of stress-related syndromes.

CHAPTER 3:

More Detailed Symptoms of Adrenal Fatigue

If you're feeling rundown and tired and seem to have a reduced tolerance for stress, the following signs and symptoms, described in more detail, can help you recognize if it may be adrenal fatigue. A definitive diagnosis of any illness must come through a licensed medical professional.

Monitor how well you tolerate and spring back from "stressors."

While many people believe stress is always a mental side effect from too much negative anguish or mentally struggling with problems, stress is actually anything that places extra demands on the mind or body. Stress can be either positive or negative and can still result in taxing both the mind and body by lowering energy reserves supplied by the adrenal glands.

Some people refer to this as being "stressed out" and while most people experience infrequent episodes of being stressed out, if it becomes chronic from being experienced either too often or for extended periods of time, the adrenal glands may begin to diminish in their ability to help the body to cope and spring back from stressors.

The adrenal glands, two small pyramid-shaped glands that sit on top of each our two kidneys, give us these stress-coping abilities via the release of a hormone they produce called "cortisol." Many medical sources call cortisol "the stress hormone" but if the adrenal glands are overextended from relentless stress placed upon them over time, the reserves of this hormone can diminish somewhat and this leaves the mind and body less able to cope with stress. This is also why adrenal fatigue is referred to as "Low Adrenal Reserve" and "Adrenal Exhaustion."

Notice your Diet Habits - Cravings for Sugary and/or Salty Foods and Stimulants

According to many sources that address adrenal fatigue, when the adrenal glands are working at sub-normal (low) levels, the body may crave more foods containing salt and sugar because these substances will raise blood pressure and energy levels, when the adrenal glands have a diminished ability to do so. The body begins to seek ways to replace the missing energy that is usually supplied in more adequate levels by the adrenal glands. Some adrenal fatigue sufferers will also crave other stimulants, such as caffeine, alcohol and tobacco or anything that helps give them a lift in their energy levels.

The problem with this scenario of stimulant-use is that the extra stimulants will usually only act to stress the adrenals even more and will result in slowed recovery from adrenal fatigue or a worsening of it over time. The stimulants will give the person using them a temporary energy-high but will be followed by a crash of more severe fatigue once the effects have worn off.

This can create a vicious cycle of highs and lows and can also result in the adrenal fatigue sufferer having more and more dependency on stimulants, to the point that they cannot get going upon waking in the mornings without a stimulant boost (i.e. a cup of coffee) nor can they get through the entire day without repeated use of them.

If you have low stress tolerance, plus find yourself craving stimulants, including more sugary and salty foods, you may have adrenal fatigue.

Watch for Physical Signs or Changes in your Body

People suffering adrenal fatigue will find that their bodies react differently to physical exertion. Physical exercise may become more difficult for them and they may find they do not tolerate it as well and may also take longer to recover from even mild to moderate physical exertion. Some adrenal fatigue sufferers will also experience mild joint and muscle aches and a vague feeling of being ill or just not feeling well.

They may also experience a condition known as "Orthostatic Hypotension," which is a slightly diminished ability by the adrenal glands to help regulate blood pressure upon standing up from a sitting or lying-down (supine) position. This condition results in blood pressure not rising as much as it normally should upon standing (in order to move the blood upward to the heart and brain). Because of this, the person will feel dizzy for a few seconds or even faint upon standing, as if they could possibly black out.

One might also feel a pressure-type sensation in their head and neck area during an episode of Orthostatic Hypotension, which is actually caused a lack of blood pressure but gives the sensation that there is extra pressure for a few seconds. There is a medical test for detecting this condition as well, called the "tilt-table test", which consists of taking a patient's blood pressure and heart rate readings, when sitting or lying flat, then again when at various upright positions.

I – the author personally have this type of dysautonomia and it would be revealed clearly if I were to have the tilt-table test done.

You can perform a home-version of this test yourself using a BP monitor, by first taking a reading while sitting, then again immediately upon standing. When I conduct this test at home, my BP drops a good 20 points and my heart rate increases 30 or more BPM. This is too much of a fluctuation and an overreaction by the involuntary nervous system, which would also be revealed via a tilt-table test and points to an involuntary nervous system that is struggling to regulate these bodily functions (dysregulated-autonomic "dys-autonomia"). If you are found to have dysautonomia, low adrenal function can be the cause and correction of the adrenal fatigue may resolve this symptom as well as the others that have been previously listed.

Some adrenal fatigue patients have also reported that they have increased sensitivity to bright light and loud sounds and can become more irritable or jumpy in the presence of these or other physical stimuli. A combination of low stress tolerance, craving stimulants and having diminished ability to handle physical activity or stimuli, can all point to the possibility of a person having adrenal fatigue.

CHAPTER 4:

Getting Tested for Adrenal Fatigue

Testing is important for determining whether a person has adrenal fatigue, in my opinion. I mention this because though it takes physical symptoms such as the ones previously described before a person will even want to investigate what could be wrong with them, getting the adrenal hormone levels tested is the single best indicator for adrenal fatigue and may also serve to rule the condition out.

The two hormones most commonly tested to determine a person's adrenal function are "cortisol and DHEA." These two hormones are the best indicators of how well the adrenal glands are functioning. Relatively inexpensive home, "saliva tests" are available to test these hormones and they are available online through a number of companies and are also carried by many pharmacies nationwide.

Saliva testing of adrenal hormones is recognized as being as reliable and accurate as blood testing by medical research groups, including the U.S. National Institutes of Health - National Library of Medicine (PubMed). If adrenal hormones are found to be low in range (normal values-reference range) or even fall slightly below the normal range, this is a more definite sign of adrenal fatigue. A result that is actually flagged clinically low should be shown to a doctor.

Keep in mind as stated earlier, that many Doctors do not recognize adrenal fatigue but will only recognize the severe type of adrenal hypo-function, called Addison's Disease. Because of this, they will believe that a patient who passes a test called the ATCH Stimulation Test, which is designed to detect full blown adrenal insufficiency, needs no further investigation however, adrenal fatigue is sub-clinical (milder) and yet can still result in serious symptoms. A patient with adrenal fatigue, will pass this test, in most cases but what they actually need tested for, are the "free levels" of the major adrenal hormones - "DHEA and Cortisol".

The ACTH Stimulation Test is designed to gauge the adrenals reaction to being stimulated by the pituitary hormone ACTH, the problem is however, that with adrenal fatigue, the adrenals can be stimulated and will react but they still produce low levels of adrenal hormones consistently and they usually crash afterward from the extra stimulation because adrenal reserves are low. Being stimulated chemically from the outside as opposed having ongoing reserves, are not the same thing.

I receive e-mails often from people who suspect they might be suffering from Adrenal Fatigue and they will relate this suspicion to their Doctors. Their Doctors will usually order them a blood test of their blood cortisol level and these patients will ask me if I feel this is a good test for Adrenal Fatigue or Adrenal Insufficiency. I usually express to them that in my opinion, blood testing needs to be the one called the "ACTH Stimulation Test", also called the "Cortrosyn Stimulation Test", which can rule out or confirm true Adrenal

Insufficiency but I also point out to them that saliva testing done at multiple times during a 24 hour period, can also detect a low or abnormal cortisol rhythm as well, such as that which manifests with adrenal fatigue. I will also mention to them that a single blood draw of cortisol levels is like a snapshot reading and doesn't actually establish how well the cortisol rhythm is functioning throughout the day.

A single blood draw, of cortisol doesn't really establish what the cortisol rhythm is doing throughout the day. A better test of adrenal function in general is the "ACTH Stimulation Test" as previously mentioned, which takes a baseline reading then two more at thirty minute intervals, after giving the patient an injection of the ACTH hormone to stimulate cortisol production. This is done to see if there is a significant increase in cortisol with the two stimulated readings and if there isn't an adequate response, they may diagnose adrenal insufficiency.

There are also saliva cortisol tests available that can help to establish a normal or abnormal cortisol circadian rhythm. These test kits contain tubes for collecting saliva samples at 3 or 4 different times during a 24 hour period. These are not terribly expensive and far less expensive than an ACTH Stimulation Test which may not be of concern if one has medical insurance that covers this type of diagnostic testing. Many pharmacies carry the saliva test kits, usually the "ZRT Labs, Inc." brand, so one can check with their local pharmacy for these. If they do not carry them, ZRT tests are also available for ordering online.

These are the reasons I believe saliva cortisol testing is the best method for detecting adrenal fatigue, once a patient has had full-blown adrenal insufficiency ruled out via an ACTH Stimulation test – should they first wish to take this precaution.

CHAPTER 5:

My Personal Struggle with Adrenal Fatigue

My own ongoing battle with adrenal fatigue began to manifest several years before I experienced the onset of hypothyroidism, caused by Hashimoto's thyroiditis in early year-2003. I began to notice months previous to diagnosis of the thyroid disorder that my tolerance for stress and my recuperative abilities, to spring back from hard physical activity, illnesses, excessive stressors etc.., was slowly diminishing to a severely depleted level. When my hypothyroidism manifested, the adrenal fatigue hit a peak of severity and the combination of the two really threw me for a loop.

The first doctors I visited did not investigate to find the thyroid disease and I was not being treated for it, so in the mean time I had to push myself incredibly hard just to keep going because I also had an extremely stressful job situation, in property management at that time and my thyroid symptoms were seriously adding to that stress.

Finally at one point, the adrenal fatigue turned into severe "adrenal exhaustion" and I experienced a strange viral-type illness that left me with a severe case of hives (these resolved over time) and swollen neck lymph-nodes that are still mildly swollen to this day. This is also the point at which my chemical sensitivities became much worse to caffeine, chocolate, alcohol and stimulants of any kind. In other words I had developed increased multiple chemical sensitivities (MCS).

I finally demanded blood tests and as a result, was treated for diagnosed hypothyroidism but the adrenal fatigue remained, re-occurring in flares of intermittent symptoms. Over time, I learned the difference between the symptoms of adrenal fatigue/exhaustion and thyroid symptoms. With adrenal exhaustion, I experience severe post-exertion malaise that can take a couple of days to recuperate from, especially after hard physical activity. My low adrenal hormone levels were confirmed through saliva and urinary testing, which revealed consistently low cortisol.

I have since been treated for these health disorders and have seen significant improvement in them. I do still experience flares of adrenal fatigue symptoms, if I venture outside of a diet restricting stimulants or if I do not keep my stress levels under control.

It is my belief that CFS is strongly associated with a type of adrenal exhaustion and that adrenal fatigue can be a forerunner to it in some cases. The most well-established feature of CFS that you find in medical research (also true of fibromyalgia), are "low cortisol levels" and I do not believe this is a coincidence but something that makes sense because the main purposes of cortisol are regulating stress and controlling inflammatory responses in the body. Two of the doctors I have been treated by since 2003, also diagnosed me with co-morbid CFS.

The adrenals when low functioning, cause more allergy, viral and illness responses to occur, due to the adrenals role in immune system function, being greatly diminished.

Cortisol is also our body's natural anti-inflammatory and so low levels give rise to joint and muscle pain and other inflammatory reactions in the body. All of these factors combined, contribute to the symptoms of adrenal fatigue and CFS and can add to the symptom struggles of hypothyroid patients who have these co-morbid conditions.

The fact is, adrenal fatigue can be a factor in these and other chronic diseases and syndromes or not be related to anything specific otherwise.

It is important when one feels they may have adrenal fatigue, to be tested for it because other hormone imbalances and illnesses cause similar symptoms. More pharmacies are now carrying "ZRT Labs" saliva hormone kits, including ones that test adrenal as well as the sex hormone levels.

The passion I have in the area of adrenal fatigue, besides having it myself, as part of CFS and co morbid to thyroid disease comes from the fact that far too many studies and reputable organizations recognize it.

This includes the "Fibro & Fatigue Centers", located in 15 states, that are staffed by Board Certified MDs from just about every field of medicine. Too many of these type sources confirm its existence and yet it is still believed to be simply a pseudo-syndrome or a psychosomatic one by some in the medical community. The fact is that there are also U.S. Government health studies concluding that there are low-cortical syndromes and well established sub-clinical forms of adrenal hypo-function, that could all be referred-to under the term; "adrenal fatigue".

CHAPTER 6:

Treatment for Adrenal Fatigue

If you test your adrenal hormones and find that they are consistently low-normal, near borderline or even clinically low, then it would be time to check into adrenal support, first through your Doctor who will first want to test to make sure you are not experiencing full-blown adrenal insufficiency. If it is found to be the milder adrenal fatigue and not actual adrenal disease causing a more severe type of adrenal insufficiency but your Doctor does not believe in treating this lesser form, you might try finding an Osteopath or Naturopath Physician, who does recognize adrenal fatigue and the treatments that are available for it.

If these avenues for treatment by a physician are not available, you may want to purchase the over-the-counter adrenal support supplements to treat the condition yourself. Should you do this, I would of course recommend taking only the manufacturer's recommended doses and that you also do some research on the support supplements you may choose to take.

This would be a wise precaution, to make sure they are safe for you and that there are no contraindications that might affect you meaning; they will not interact negatively with any other treatments you may already be taking for other health issues.

Following the subheading below, are methods and treatments that can help to improve adrenal fatigue and to possibly resolve it over time.

Get more Sleep, Rest and Relaxation

In today's fast-paced society, a busy schedule can leave little time for adequate sleep, rest and relaxation. This lack of rest can heighten your stress level and place too much demand on the adrenal glands. Like any organ or gland of the body, the adrenals need time to rest and recuperate in order to rebuild their reserves and abilities to function at optimal level. The job of these glands is to supply the body with adequate levels of adrenal hormones, but they can only do this if the body in general is allowed to rest and relax for sufficient periods of time each day.

Medical sources state that most people need a minimum of eight hours of sleep per night in order to function at their best level during the daytime and in order for the cells of the body to have adequate time to repair and restore from normal use of them. Our everyday routines also place a degree of stress upon our minds and emotions. While sleep is very important to get in adequate amounts, the same is true of simple rest and relaxation in general. If you don't allow for necessary leisure time and time to simply sit quietly or lie down and rest on occasion, you will not be allowing your body and mind to unwind from the stressors of everyday duties and this leads to that feeling of being "stressed out" by the end of the day or even before the end of the day.

Reduce your Stress Levels

No one living in the world today can escape or be immune to stress. Stress is a fact of life; our goal is to work on reducing its effects and to learn coping skills, so that we find ways to eliminate or remove as much of it as we possibly can from our lives.

The adrenal glands help us to cope with and to recover from stress by providing the body with adequate levels of the stress hormone "cortisol" as mentioned in previous chapters. This hormone is also considered to be a "fight or flight" hormone, like adrenaline – the other major hormone released by the adrenals.

While adrenaline is the more short term energizing hormone needed at times of danger (to escape or fight a situation or enemy), cortisol is the long term fight or flight hormone, giving us the needed steady flow of energy, throughout the day, to perform our normal tasks. Relentless and ongoing stress can eventually use up the reserves of this hormone faster than the adrenals are able to supply it, unless we allow ourselves time to recuperate from stress. Only then can the adrenals rebuild the reserves of this very important stress hormone and the others it continually supplies to the body.

Stress can be reduced simply by resting and giving ourselves time during each day to unwind for a few minutes at a time.

It is also important not to become unnecessarily uptight throughout the day over small problems that arise. We should learn to not take the smaller problems as seriously, because there are potentially too many of them that can arise and this will keep our stress levels peaked too often and for extended periods of time.

Take Supplements that help Strengthen your Adrenals

There are many supplements that can be self-administered or prescribed by a qualified physician, to help keep the body and the adrenal glands healthy and strengthened to handle the everyday stress life brings upon all of us. A really good multi-vitamin is always a great idea and there are many good ones available, to choose from. Some major vitamin companies actually manufacture vitamins called "stress formulas" or "stress tabs" and these contain the vitamins and minerals that help the body cope-with and recover from stress.

Vitamin supplements in particular that are very helpful to the adrenal glands include the "B" vitamins – in particular, B-12, B-5 and B-6. Vitamin "C" is also an important vitamin for healthy adrenal function and also serves to help other vitamins absorb properly in the body. Minerals that can help with adrenal function include zinc, selenium and magnesium. There are also adrenal herbal formulas that contain helpful supplements such as "licorice root extract", "Asian ginseng" and "ashwagandha" but these should be researched carefully by anyone who is considering taking them as a short-term or long-term regimen and should also be discussed with your doctor before taking them. Purchasing supplements only from reliable, reputable companies is also wise.

Other natural supplements that can be taken to support the adrenals after observing the aforementioned precautions include "adrenal glandular" (usually beef source) and DHEA, an over-the-counter adrenal hormone that also acts as a precursor to sex hormones.

All of these supplements can potentially be helpful, but everyone is unique and some supplements work better for some people than they do for others. Sometimes it simply takes a trial of several of these, by a process of elimination, to find the one that eventually helps the most.

Use Adrenal Steroids only under Professional Supervision

Over the past few years, I've corresponded with 100s of patients who relate the fact that they suffer severe types of "Adrenal Fatigue". They report that some of their Doctors placed them on a trial of a corticosteroid drug, which is a steroid form of cortisol, to help increase their levels of this adrenal hormone that can become constantly low in people with Adrenal Fatigue. Cortisol is essential to our bodies in everyday functioning and in coping with everyday stressors as mentioned in several previous chapters but it also serves as an inflammatory agent in the body.

In Adrenal Fatigue patients, the trick in using safe non-steroid supplements, is to strengthen ones own adrenal glands, so that they function better in producing cortisol and other important adrenal hormones. With the more severe "Adrenal Insufficiency" (full blown), patients must be treated with a corticosteroid steroid, to replace the low cortisol as a lifelong treatment that cannot be substituted.

Treatment with corticosteroids requires strict doctor supervision and is especially true with that fact that some patient's cases are more complicated than others. Patients may be at risk for developing Cushings' Disease from prolonged use of adrenal steroids or may be on the verge of developing it, if they are not monitored closely. In cases like these, they may also have to be tapered off of the cortisol drug, which comes in prescribed brands such as "Cortef" and "Prednisone", very slowly and if while doing so, their cortisol drops down to adrenal insufficiency level, they may need to be bumped back up on their dose again.

These facts demonstrate the importance in a medical professional being involved, who is experienced at titrating (adjusting) the steroid dose. Some patients may also have to take the cortisol steroid for the rest of their lives, even if their adrenal insufficiency began as a mild case. Certainly this does not occur in every case of adrenal fatigue that is treated with a corticosteroid and some actually see their low adrenal function improve, so that the corticosteroid eventually elevates abnormally high in their system and will need to be discontinued. If for example, a patient develops symptoms of swelling (edema), increased appetite and weight gain while the drug is being administered, these can be symptoms of having abnormally high cortisol levels in the body, resulting in cushionoid type symptoms.

When patients are placed on corticosteroids they need follow up blood retesting and/or urine retesting of their cortisol levels, at regular intervals, similar to how thyroid hormone therapy is monitored, at two to three month intervals. If this isn't done, they can potentially develop symptoms of Cushings' Disease as previously described.

I do have a number of online articles in regard to treating Adrenal Fatigue and I don't recommend treating it with corticosteroids (cortisol steroids), whether it's the synthetic type like Prednisone or the more natural Cortef brand, unless it is a severe case that other methods and supplements have failed to improve. The reason I discourage it for cases that are only mild to moderate, is for the very reasons I have stated. Another reason steroid treatment for Adrenal Fatigue, is not recommended, is due to the possibility of it actually progressing the Adrenal Fatigue, to full blown adrenal insufficiency. This is what occurred in patients with Chronic Fatigue Syndrome who were administered cortisol drugs in trial treatment studies conducted by the U.S. National Institutes of Health.

The studies by the U.S.-NIH and by other medical research groups have found that treating sub-clinical adrenal insufficiency syndromes, such as Chronic Fatigue Syndrome and Post Traumatic Stress Disorder, can result in further adrenal suppression.

Dr. Stephen E. Straus, M.D, who is quoted in a PubMed article states; "Any time long-term steroid therapy is considered, even a low dose," he continues, "one needs to be concerned that the treatment itself may suppress the adrenal gland's normal production of steroids, which can lead to serious complications. ..." There have also been studies using smaller physiological doses that yielded promising results and that did not result in adrenal suppression in similar trials, which means it could simply be a matter of determining a safe dose level, which will hopefully be definitively determined in the near future as studies continue.

Some Doctors who do treat Adrenal Fatigue with Cortef or Prednisone, will administer it in very small physiological doses as mentioned and in so doing, can usually avoid complications, with also closely monitoring the patient's cortisol levels via repeat blood testing and by only treating them short-term until their own adrenal glands have improved. Even with this however, it carries a risk and a patient would want to be very confident in their treating Doctor.

You cannot switch from a corticosteroid also called glucocorticoids, to a simple adrenal support regimen because Adrenal Fatigue support supplements are designed to strengthen a person's own adrenal glands, so that they will begin producing their own adequate amounts of cortisol and most adrenal support, is safe enough that it can be taken lifelong, like most vitamins and minerals can.

If you are placed on a corticosteroid for Adrenal Fatigue, you'll need close supervision by your Doctor in getting better adjusted on dose or weaned off of the medication when needed. It is extremely important that you not try weaning off the medication yourself if you are being treated with the drug because this can potentially cause you to experience an "adrenal crisis", an emergency medical condition that can cause coma or death, if not treated in time.

It wasn't my intention to frighten or overly concern anyone but corticosteroid treatment is something that takes extreme caution and supervision by a Doctor and you cannot switch from such a treatment, to a different type, on your own.

The Everything Adrenal Fatigue Book

If you are not confident in your current Doctor in following through with your current treatment or in tapering you off of it, I recommend seeing another highly qualified Doctor, such as an Endocrinologist for a second opinion because corticosteroid treatment is a very serious thing and you cannot take chances with it.

Incorporate Regular Exercise into your Health Regimen

Exercise is important in strengthening the body and endocrine system in general. Regular exercise also results in strengthened adrenal glands specifically. Doctors know that exercise helps hormones in our bodies to do their job better because it helps them to circulate properly and to metabolize in the system better. Cortisol, though being the stress hormone, also helps to regulate our glucose (blood sugar) and is one reason exercise helps in this process as well.

When you begin an exercise routine, it is important that you do so at the pace your body can tolerate. You do not want to overdo on exercise, whether it is the aerobic type of those for strengthening muscles.

Too much exercise will not increase the benefit from it faster, but can actually have an adverse effect if not properly paced. This is especially true of people who are already experiencing adrenal fatigue. They can have reduced tolerance for exercise and if they do not pace themselves, they can worsen the adrenal fatigue rather than helping to resolve it.

Walking is one of the best exercises to start out with, and just a good everyday exercise for anyone. Some who start with walking can eventually progress to jogging, if that's what they chose at the proper time and pace. If you prefer walking as your exercise, many sources state that walking 15 to 20 minutes at least three times a week will give you a healthy benefit, and five times or more per week increases that benefit.

People with adrenal fatigue can incorporate these methods of lifestyle changes, diet and helpful, safe supplements into a daily regimen and can over time see significant improvement in adrenal fatigue symptoms.

Some patients may see their adrenal fatigue completely resolve over time, using these treatment suggestions, tailored to their specific needs, which can also help to decrease the chances of the adrenal - stress syndrome from returning.

SECTION TWO – (Pages 50 - 119):
The Best Darn CFS, Fibromyalgia and Adrenal
Fatigue Book!

CHAPTER 1:

Common Symptoms of Chronic Fatigue Syndrome

A Medically Recognized Illness

According to medical research and sources, Chronic Fatigue Syndrome (CFS) is characterized by its main symptom of "fatigue" not explained by another existing illness.
In order for severe, chronic fatigue to be considered as a possibility for being caused by CFS, it must be experienced for at least six months, with no significant relief during any of this time period. It is also described by medical criteria (for diagnosis) as not being relieved by sleep or rest.

People suffering CFS will find that sleep does not refresh them, even when they get adequate or more-than adequate amounts of sleep (eight hours or more).

This symptom of severe, chronic fatigue is the major, characterizing feature of CFS, including post exertional malaise (intolerance to physical exercise and exertion).

Joint and Muscle Pain

People with CFS will find that they have joint and muscle aches that are very concerning and somewhat disabling, but the joints and muscles will not swell or exhibit redness around them (as happens with different types of arthritis). These joint and muscle aches will be mild to moderate and may also cause stiffness and slightly reduced mobility.

The body aches often resemble those experienced when a person has the flu. With some CFS patients, this symptom is intermittent and with others, it is continual. If a patient has more severe and widespread body pain, along with "tender points," which are small areas where the muscle attaches to joints that are very tender to finger-point pressure, this can indicate "Fibromyalgia Syndrome" (FMS) rather than Chronic Fatigue Syndrome. These two syndromes have been found to have 75% crossover similarities.

Swollen Lymph Nodes

According to the U.S. Centers for Disease Control (CDC), "swollen lymph nodes" are also a major symptom of CFS. Those that become swollen are commonly located in the neck, just under the tonsil area on both sides, with swelling being detectable to the touch (palpation) and are also referred to as glands ("nodes" is the correct term). Lymph nodes under the armpits are also commonly found to be swollen with cases of CFS.

Medical research still has not identified the exact cause(s) of Chronic Fatigue Syndrome but some research study conclusions have shown that CFS patients commonly have high blood-titers (lab result measurements) of lifetime viruses. These lifetime viruses that affect a large percentage of the population include the "Epstein-Barr virus," which causes mononucleosis in some people who contract it.

Other people are infected by the Epstein-Barr virus without symptoms but become lifetime carriers of it.

In Chronic Fatigue Syndrome patients, these viruses might explain the flu-like symptoms they experience and the swollen lymph nodes. In people with compromised immune systems, it is believed that these viruses can replicate and reactivate. This reactivation is sometimes referred-to as "post viral illness".

Co-morbid Adrenal Fatigue

It has also been found that CFS patients have less ability to cope with and recover from stress. Medical research, including that conducted by the U.S. National Institutes of Health, has found that CFS patients are low in an adrenal hormone called "cortisol." This is the "stress hormone" and studies have concluded that the low adrenal function in CFS patients might be due to an altered "hypothalamic-pituitary-adrenal axis" (HPA Axis), which is a term to describe the three endocrine glands that regulate adrenal function and work in sync with each other to supply proper levels of the cortisol hormone.

It is theorized that the function of these glands becomes "blunted" (reduced) in CFS patients, resulting in reduced adrenal cortisol levels. Researchers do not know at this point if the low cortisol (adrenal fatigue) is a cause or a result of CFS, but they do believe it is a factor that contributes to its symptoms. A person who suspects they may have adrenal fatigue or CFS can purchase home saliva tests kits at their local pharmacy, or online, to determine if their adrenal hormones are low.

Multiple Chemical Sensitivities

In addition to the other symptoms addressed in the previous subheadings, many CFS sufferers also find that they have become sensitive to many different chemicals that they were not previously intolerant to. They may find that certain household cleaners, perfumes, deodorants, etc. cause them different types of allergic reactions or sensitivity symptoms.

This can also be true of certain foods or drinks that were not a problem before the onset of the syndrome but can be especially true of stimulants such as caffeine, chocolate and alcohol.

The Everything Adrenal Fatigue Book

These chemical sensitivities can trigger CFS symptoms when patients with the syndrome come in contact with them or consume them.

Neurological Symptoms

People with Chronic Fatigue Syndrome may also find that they experience headaches of a different or unusual type and/or neurological-type pain sensations. These headaches and body aches may be described as nerve-type pains and that headaches seem to radiate to other nerves within the body.

These types of nerve-related pains are sometimes referred to as "peripheral neuropathy" and can be found in other illnesses in addition to CFS, including diabetes and thyroid diseases.

Nerve-related sensations in CFS patients can include tingling and numbness in the extremities (hands and feet).

Neurological symptoms can also include "Neurally Mediated Hypotension," a condition that results in blood pressure becoming irregular, especially upon first standing from a seated position, also referred to as "Orthostatic Hypotension" and "Postural Hypotension". When a CFS patient experiences this neurological symptom, they may feel dizzy and/or faint upon rising after sitting or lying down (from supine positions).

Ruling Out Other Illnesses

If other underlying medical conditions have been ruled-out as a cause of CFS symptoms, through complete and thorough blood testing and other medical lab tests, this can help point to a diagnosis of CFS. When patients with the previously-described symptoms are thoroughly checked by their doctors and have had a complete battery of tests to rule out all possible causes, this gives a much stronger case for a diagnosis of Chronic Fatigue Syndrome.

There are many illnesses and diseases that can present with the same (or similar) symptoms of CFS but medical blood-lab tests and other diagnostic procedures that can confirm or rule out these other illnesses. Should a patient complete such testing and be found to be "negative" for all other causes, this is the single most definitive way to confirm that a patient's symptoms are caused by CFS, rather than another underlying medical condition.

Interesting Facts about CFS

According to reputable medical sources, Chronic Fatigue Syndrome does not typically cause organ damage and is not a fatal illness, although there are disagreements and varied opinions in this regard. Studies of the syndrome have found that some patients recover from CFS within two to five years of experiencing the onset of it, while other patients may have the illness for many years or throughout their lives.

Symptom-flares of CFS can be intermittent with varied changes in the severity of them with each episode or in some patients may remain severe and ongoing.

Other interesting facts about CFS include the following:

- CFS affects over 1-million people in the U.S. alone.
- CFS is from 3 to 4 times as common in women as in men.
- CFS affects more people in their 40s and 50s than in other age groups.
- CFS is rare in childhood and adolescence, with teenagers being the most affected youth-group.
- CFS is more commonly referred-to as Myalgic Encephalomyelitis (ME) in the UK.

There are treatments that help to reduce the symptoms of CFS and that can help patients regain a better quality of life. Those who are diagnosed with this serious but treatable syndrome should discuss the available treatment-options with their doctors.

CHAPTER 2:

The Suspected Causes of CFS

Triggers for Chronic Fatigue Syndrome

Decades of medical research on Chronic Fatigue
Syndrome has revealed a number of abnormalities
in patients with the syndrome. One definitive
cause has yet to be found.
Chronic Fatigue Syndrome (CFS) is a
complicated and sometimes mysterious illness.
Medical research studies have been ongoing for
many years in attempts to find a definitive cause
for the illness. Medical groups studying CFS have
instead found a number of aspects of the
syndrome that are clearly present but each may
play a role or be one of the many factors of CFS
rather than its definitive cause.

Post Viral Illness

A number of viruses studied in relation to CFS
have been found to be present in significant titers
(lab result measurements) in people suffering the
syndrome.

Among the viruses suspected of being possible causes or triggers for CFS, are enteroviruses and retroviruses. These include the Epstein-Barr Virus (EBV) that is usually contracted during childhood and carried throughout one's lifetime, human herpesvirus 6 and the Cytomegalovirus. Candida albican overgrowth (fungal/yeast infection), although not in the virus category has also been suspected as a possible cause or trigger for CFS.

Some of these viruses, including EBV cause no symptoms in most people when contracted (can potentially cause mononucleosis) but will increase in the number of titers found in the blood when the virus replicates. It has been proposed as a possibility that the increased replication of viruses may occur when the immune system is not functioning well in suppressing their ability to replicate or reactivate. Reactivation would mean that a virus resurges at times, causing repeated illness in the infected person who has not fully developed immunity to it.

Imbalance in the Involuntary Nervous System

In other studies of CFS patients, they have been found to be experiencing dysfunction in their involuntary nervous systems (INS), also referred to as "autonomic failure" and "dysautonomia". The INS is responsible for regulating blood pressure with changes in physical activity and changes in positions of the body (i.e. sitting, standing and lying flat). It also regulates all other involuntary bodily functions, including respiration, digestion, kidney function, liver function, etc… and increases these functions when needed (sympathetic response) or decreases them (parasympathetic response).

An imbalance in this system will cause these functions to be inadequate at times and over-responsive at other times. If for example, physical activity is increased and blood pressure needs to rise but fails to do so, this can result in bodily fatigue due to a lack of needed blood flow to the muscles and organs of the body. If bodily functions need to decrease at times of rest or when sleep is needed but remain highly activated this will result in fatigue as well.

Dysfunction of the Immune System

Other, conclusions resulting from medical studies of CFS causes, have found that patients with the syndrome are experiencing a dysfunction of the immune system. The immunity or what might be referred to as "resistance" to viruses and allergens is greatly diminished in CFS patients. This means that the body is more susceptible to viruses and allergens and recovers more slowly from exposure and infections to them, than are people with healthy immune systems.

Infections of these types can cause a mild systemic (system-wide) inflammation in the body and cause the person experiencing them, to feel as if they are experiencing perpetual flu-like symptoms or a continual low-grade fever.

Chronic Stress

CFS patients often report in medical study questionnaires that they experienced severe, prolonged or traumatic stress, just before the onset of their CFS symptoms.

Stress is responded-to by the part of the endocrine system called the "HPA Axis", standing for the Hypothalamus-Pituitary-Adrenal gland system. When chronic stress is experienced, this system is hyper-active and over time, becomes "blunted", meaning it becomes fatigued or diminished in its ability to run at overdrive. This causes slower release of the hormones that come from these endocrine glands that work in sync (full-circle) to supply the body with stress coping abilities.

The end result of the hypothalamus stimulating the pituitary gland, which then in-turn stimulates the adrenal glands, is the release of the stress hormone "cortisol". When this system becomes blunted after extended hyperactivity, cortisol levels begin to fall or what is sometimes referred to as "hypocortisolemia" or "hypoadrenia". Some sources recognizing this mild form of adrenal dysfunction refer to it as "Adrenal Fatigue".

CHAPTER 3:

More on Dysautonomia in Chronic Fatigue Syndrome

CFS and the Involuntary Nervous System

There are many associated causes of Chronic Fatigue Syndrome but one of the more significant connections is imbalance in the involuntary nervous system – "dysautonomia".

People with Chronic Fatigue Syndrome (CFS) have been found in research studies, to be experiencing imbalances in their involuntary nervous systems (INS) or "autonomic failure". This part of the nervous system is responsible for increasing bodily functions when needed (sympathetic) and decreasing them when needed (parasympathetic). The bodily functions affected by the INS include blood pressure, heart rate, breathing, bodily fluid balance and digestion.

Imbalances in the INS also called the "autonomic nervous system" is sometimes referred to by the medical term "dysautonomia".

The Everything Adrenal Fatigue Book

While strong association between dysfunction of the INS in patients with CFS has been clearly established, there is still no definitive explanation as to why this connection exists or as to whether the problems with the INS are a cause of CFS or a result of it. It is clear however that dysautonomia plays a significant role in the symptom-complex of CFS.

Orthostatic Hypotension-Dizziness upon Standing

One of the more common forms of dysautonomia experienced by CFS patients is called "Orthostatic Hypotension" (OH). This condition causes the blood pressure to drop with positional changes of the body but occurs more often when a person is rising from a seated or lying down position (supine) to a standing position. It is also referred to as "postural hypotension" and some medical sources refer to it as "neurally mediated hypotension".

Normally, blood pressure rises slightly when a person first stands up, which allows blood to be transferred from the lower part of the body, to the upper part of the body.

With orthostatic hypotension the blood pressure instead will drop slightly, causing a person to feel lightheaded, dizzy, headachy and faint. Some people with this condition do actually pass out but is not common. Because of this abnormal and sudden drop in blood pressure, some people with OH will also experience a short term increase in heart rate, referred to as "tachycardia" (beats exceeding 100 per minute without exertion). This is the body's attempt to correct the sudden episode of hypotension.

Postural Orthostatic Tachycardia Syndrome (POTS) and CFS

POTS, is a form of dysautonomia that is diagnosed by neurologists and other physicians who specialize in nervous system disorders. When symptoms of OH and tachycardia are serious enough and result in other significant symptoms, a diagnosis of POTS may be given. Some medical research groups are finding that the similarities between POTS and CFS may point to these syndromes as being one and the same in some patients, rather than being two separate illnesses.

If this is proven to be the case at some point, CFS may be placed in the category of neurological illness. While post viral illness and other proposed factors are also being studied as causes of CFS, the resulting effect on the nervous system may prove to be the most significant factor in the syndrome.

Treatments for Dysautonomia

Dysautonomia and CFS are also similar in the fact that both illnesses have no specific treatments available for them. There are effective treatments to control or to relieve symptoms of these illnesses but each patient experiences the varied symptoms of these syndromes to different degrees. Some patients may be treated with beta-blocker medications that help control blood pressure and heart rate irregularities.

Others may be treated with drugs that control neurological symptoms such as those used to treat epilepsy while others may be treated with mineral corticosteroids (mineral version of cortisol steroid) that helps regulate blood pressure.

Yet others may be prescribed psychiatric medications to help them cope with the severity of symptoms that can impact emotions or Cognitive Behavioral Therapy that helps them cope psychologically with their syndromes.

CHAPTER 4:

Common Symptoms and Diagnosis of Fibromyalgia

The Syndrome of Widespead and Chronic Muscle Pain

Fibromyalgia is a syndrome of widespread body pain and fatigue. There are signs and symptoms that can help to identify and diagnose fibromyalgia.

People with fibromyalgia syndrome (FMS) will find that they experience widespread and severe body pain that is chronic (ongoing). The pain will affect the muscles and joints but will also produce "tender points." These are places on the body that experience pain when pressure is applied to them, where muscles are attached to bones, at the joints. Some in the medical community vary in their opinions as to whether FMS is a rheumatic condition or strictly a pain syndrome. Others believe it is a combination of both.

Diagnostic Criteria for Fibromyalgia

In addition to also being recognized as an inflammatory disorder, some research studies have also found that FMS may be an autoimmune-related disorder. Some medical research groups have also found that FMS and Chronic Fatigue Syndrome (CFS) have 75% crossover symptom similarities.

Some published diagnostic studies have suggested that fibromyalgia is better determined when a person experiencing FMS symptoms is found to have at least 11 of the 18 possible tender points that can occur throughout the body. These are areas where pain will occur upon applying mild pressure to them, using a fingertip.

The areas on the body where these tender points may occur include the following:

- the hips
- the knees
- the back of the head near the base of the neck
- upper areas of the chest
- the upper back in the cervical spine area
- the elbows
- the shoulders

Fatigue and Sleep Disturbances

Fatigue is another major symptom of FMS and it is sometimes exacerbated by sleep disturbances that can also occur. The fatigue is often relentless and proper sleep and rest does little to alleviate it completely. Normal circadian sleep rhythms (cycles) that are supposed to occur become abnormal in fibromyalgia patients, which results in daytime sleepiness and feeling more awake during nighttime hours.

Medical research, including that conducted by the National Institutes of Health (U.S.-NIH), suggests that abnormal functioning of the adrenal glands is one possible cause of the disrupted sleep patterns, due to the adrenal hormone "cortisol" not being properly regulated by the adrenal glands in people who have fibromyalgia.

Digestive Disturbances and IBS

FMS patients may complain of severe indigestion, heartburn and acid reflux with FMS but may also experience alternating spells of constipation and diarrhea. This may indicate that they are also suffering from Irritable Bowel Syndrome (IBS). Frequent gastritis and bloating may also manifest as part of the digestive problems that can occur with fibromyalgia.

Headaches and Sensory Disturbances

Many people with fibromyalgia experience frequent headaches and these may have a neurological aspect to them that they have not experienced previously.

The headaches may sometimes have an unusual pattern to them or will affect the person's senses as they occur (i.e. eyesight, sense of smell, taste and hearing). These sensory changes can occur with headaches or may also occur without them.

These may include heightened and/or loss of sensitivity to the following:

• light
• noises
• flavors
• odors
• sense of touch

Emotional and Mental Symptoms

People with FMS may also experience symptoms of anxiety and depression and a change in mental functioning. These emotional symptoms may alternate between those of anxiety and depression or the patient may experience mostly one of these mood problems. A person with fibromyalgia may experience anxiety symptoms as an increase in chronic worry and episodes of fear, including the possibility of panic attacks.

The depression may be perceived by them as a profound sadness, an emptiness or hopelessness.

This demonstrates the importance in monitoring fibromyalgia patients for any signs of worsening emotional symptoms, which may require treatment as a separate issue, in addition to treatments that are needed for rheumatic symptoms (muscle pain).

Mental functioning may also become diminished in fibromyalgia patients. They may have difficulty concentrating and will experience what is often referred to as "brain fog," a term to describe mental dullness or an inability to focus with the same sharpness they had previous to their illness. Short-term memory loss is also experience in some FMS patients.

See Your Doctor

People who experience the symptoms described in the subheadings above need to see a qualified, licensed medial physician in order to confirm a diagnosis of fibromyalgia or other conditions with similar symptoms. Patients receiving a diagnosis of FMS can move forward with appropriate treatment, which can help to control symptoms or diminish them significantly and return them to an improved quality of life.

CHAPTER 5:

Common Causes of Adrenal Fatigue Syndrome

Conditions that Contribute to Exhausted Adrenals

Adrenal Fatigue may be the most common health condition that exists. Chronic stressors, lack of rest and sleep and other illnesses can all be factors in this syndrome.

Some Adrenal Fatigue sources state that there are several stages of altered adrenal function that occur before the glands become exhausted. These include a stage when the glands are hyper-active or what might be referred to as the "alarm stage", followed by a "resistance stage" in which the adrenals withdraw from completing full day cycles of stress coping and finally, they reach a fatigued state in which stress-coping is greatly diminished. If the Adrenal Fatigue stage is not treated and reversed, complete adrenal exhaustion can also be experienced.

Mental and Emotional Stressors

Ongoing chronic stress from work, school and problems in life that might arise can place added mental and emotional pressures on a person causing a draining effect on their adrenal reserves. The hormones produced by the adrenal glands will be in greater demand in these type circumstances and although they can meet that demand for reasonable periods of time, if severe and prolonged stressors continue, this ability becomes diminished over time. The main hormone affected by this syndrome is "cortisol" that supplies the body with stress-coping and recovery abilities and supplies the body with steady energy as it also aids in glucose regulation (blood sugar).

Physical Stressors

Overextending one's physical limitations over long periods of time can contribute to reduced adrenal function as well. Continually working extended shifts on a job for example that leaves a person physically exhausted would be an example of a chronic physical stressor.

Athletes that undergo strenuous training have been studied in medical research and found to experience significant, short-term increases in cortisol levels (alarm stage). Not getting proper rest to help the body recover from physical activity is also a factor in cortisol regulation.

Another example of physical stressors, are chronic diseases and illnesses that seriously affect energy levels in the body. These add physical demands on the body due to the fact that in spite of illness, people are often required to carry on the same duties and responsibilities they had before contracting their illnesses. Inflammatory diseases can be especially taxing on adrenal function because inflammation is also responded to by the cortisol hormone which is the body's natural anti-inflammatory. Cancer patients commonly experience varied degrees of adrenal insufficiency as a result of both the disease and its treatments.

Lack of Sleep

During sleep, the adrenal glands have opportunity to recharge hormone reserves.

Studies of sleep and wake cycles and their effects on adrenal hormone levels have shown that inadequate sleep can seriously affect the cortisol circadian rhythm during waking hours. An adequate number of hours for deep sleep or what is also referred to as REM-sleep (rapid eye movement stage) are required for 24 hour cortisol cycles to complete appropriately. Lack of sleep or broken sleep patterns (fragmented) can contribute to symptoms of adrenal fatigue or can be a direct cause of it. Other research studies have shown that sleep deprivation can also cause symptoms similar to those of Chronic Fatigue Syndrome and Fibromyalgia.

Excessive use of Stimulants

When a person is experiencing a lack of energy, he may resort to increased use of stimulants to get them through the day. Stimulants increase adrenal hormone levels, including adrenaline and cortisol but can also cause these hormones to drop afterward as the stimulant diminishes from the body.

This can cause a vicious cycle of highs and lows and an increase in stimulant use, which can also advance to use of drugs or alcohol as a means to cope with downward fluctuations in energy levels. Some people become stimulant-dependent to the point of not being able to start their day without the use of one.

These scenarios occur commonly to millions of people in the U.S. and worldwide. It has in fact been suggested by some sources that adrenal fatigue may be the most common illness affecting the population in this stressful age we live in. Some statistics state that the syndrome may affect as much as 80% of the population at some point in their lives but treatments are available that help reduce symptoms and in some cases may completely resolve the illness.

CHAPTER 6:

Adrenal Fatigue or Adrenal Insufficiency?

Mild vs Full Blown Adrenal Hypofunctioning

Adrenal Fatigue is a mild form of adrenal insufficiency affecting the rhythm of the adrenal glands rather than their ability to function normally when less fatigued.

More medical doctors from all areas of practice are recognizing the syndrome known as "Adrenal Fatigue" than at any time in the past. Years of reluctance for many of them, in accepting this common stress syndrome as a real illness, came from the fact that the condition is less-than full blown adrenal insufficiency. The diagnostic testing used to diagnose Adrenal fatigue, is often not as black and white or definitive as that used to diagnose true adrenal insufficiency. If however, it can be diagnosed, treatments are available.

Adrenal Function Testing

The test most often used to diagnose adrenal insufficient states, which are often placed in the Addison's disease category (acute adrenocortical failure) is the "ACTH Stimulation" test, also referred to as the "Cortrosyn Stimulation Test". The test is administered by injecting the testee/patient with ACTH (adrenocorticotropic hormone) which, is the hormone normally sent from the pituitary gland in the brain, to stimulate the adrenal glands to produce cortisol.

This hormone also called "cortical", is the body's stress-coping hormone that gives the body recuperative abilities to handle daily stressors and to recover from traumatic or severe stress-inducing events. Once injected, the testee's cortisol level is monitored to see if it rises adequately, in response to being stimulated by ACTH. If the response by the adrenals is non-existent or weak, a diagnosis of adrenal insufficiency may be given as a result.

Adrenal Rhythm

With Adrenal Fatigue, the ACTH Stimulation test will usually result in a normal reading because the issue with the syndrome is not whether the adrenals can be stimulated to produce cortisol but whether they can maintain the level of cortisol in a steady rhythm as needed by the body.

Adrenal Fatigue is also referred to as a condition of "low adrenal reserve", meaning the adrenals can at times function at normal or sub-normal levels but cannot complete full daily cycles of supplying cortisol to the body as it is needed. This leaves the person's body in a stressed-out state at the end of a day of coping with stressors.

At some stages of Adrenal Fatigue, cortisol can peak at times the body needs it less, such as at times of rest or sleep when less stress-coping is needed. Adversely, the cortisol reserve may become low at active times during the day when stress-coping is needed the most.

The Role of Stress in Adrenal Fatigue

One term used in describing Adrenal Fatigue, is to refer to it as a syndrome of "stressed adrenals". The symptoms of diminished stress-coping include fatigue, nervousness, depression, irritability, the need for stimulants and a low tolerance for stressors of any kind. The syndrome often manifests in people who have experienced traumatic events (Post Traumatic Stress Disorder) or chronic stress, meaning unrelenting, prolonged and severe. It often also manifests in people with chronic diseases, including thyroid conditions, diabetes, cancer and autoimmune diseases of all types.

Adrenal Fatigue has been cited in many medical research studies, as playing a major role in conditions such as Chronic Fatigue Syndrome, Fibromyalgia and Post traumatic Stress Disorder. While the condition is not referred to as Adrenal Fatigue in these research studies, it is fully described as a condition of "mild adrenal insufficiency" and as "hypocortisolemia", among other terms.

CHAPTER 7:

The Accuracy of Saliva Adrenal Cortisol Testing

How does Saliva Cortisol Compare to Blood Levels?

The development of saliva test kits for measuring adrenal hormones has proven to be an accurate and convenient method of in-home testing for detecting mild forms of adrenal hypo-function.

Cortisol, the major adrenal hormone also called "cortical" is the most important hormone level tested, to determine how well the adrenal glands are functioning. Each person has two glands, each sitting directly on top of a kidney gland, located on both sides of the lower back. The glands are small, being about the size of a grape but are responsible for the body's ability to survive, cope-with and recover from stress, including everyday stressors and those that are traumatic or severe.

The adrenals also produce hormones that are precursors to sex hormones, meaning the initial hormones produced by the glands will convert into other hormones, including the sex ones, as needed in the body.

More Adrenal Testing Options are Now Available

With the emergence of recognition for mild to moderate levels of adrenal insufficiency, often referred to as "Adrenal Fatigue" or "Adrenal Exhaustion", more testing options have been developed for testing adrenal function. In addition to the test for detecting full blown adrenal insufficiency called the "ACTH Stimulation test", other tests to detect abnormal adrenal function, including those that help detect overactive adrenal glands (Cushing's syndrome) have become increasingly available in recent years. These tests include collecting urine samples over a 24 hour period, to determine adrenal cortisol output and saliva samples that can be collected at different times of the day to establish the rhythm of cortisol output.

Medical Research says Saliva Cortisol Tests are Accurate

Medical groups that have studied adrenal-cortisol testing by saliva samples, have determined this type testing to be accurate, as well as less intrusive and more convenient than blood sampling. Mention is also made in these studies that multiple levels can be obtained at different points of a full day-cycle (24 hour period) which would be difficult to accomplish by blood sampling.

Saliva samples can be done in the convenience of a person's home while multiple blood draws would require long stays or repeated visits to blood draw clinics when taking multiple samples during a 24-hour period. When citing conclusions on saliva testing to detect Cushing's syndrome, the Journal of Clinical Endocrinology & Metabolism states that it is as accurate as plasma measurements and better than urineglucocorticoid excretion.

Salivary Cortisol Measurements

Saliva Test Kits are available online and through Pharmacies. Consumers, who wish to test their adrenal function in the privacy of their homes, can now purchase saliva test kits that accurately measure both cortisol and DHEA hormone levels. Many pharmacies are now carrying kits by reputable labs that analyze saliva samples, including those manufactured by ZRT Labs, Inc. and Great Smokies Diagnostic Laboratory (GSDL). These companies also offer saliva test kits to determine sex hormone levels in addition to the adrenal ones. Saliva sex hormone testing is also used by medical research groups, including World Health Organizations.

If you order testing through your pharmacy, results are returned to them, so that your pharmacist can go over the results with you. If you order test kits online, the results are sent directly to you. While this type testing requires no doctor visit, people who use them should take their results to their doctor for evaluation if abnormal results are returned or regardless of results so that it can be entered into your medical files.

CHAPTER 8:

Cortisol Supplementation for Adrenal Fatigue

Are Steroids Safe for Exhausted Adrenals?

Cortisol supplementation for chronic Adrenal Fatigue carries potential risks but may be an effective treatment if administered by a qualified, monitoring physician.

People suffering chronic Adrenal Fatigue (frequent or ongoing), will often diligently seek a treatment that will provide them relief for their concerning symptoms. For many, the option of cortisol replacement therapy is seriously considered and some patients find physicians willing to give them a trial of the treatment. Glucocorticoids, which are synthetic cortisol replacement drugs, are steroids that require caution when used to treat adrenal disorders or health conditions of any kind.

Cortisol Supplementation Requires a Qualified Physician

While some cases of Adrenal Fatigue have been successfully treated using synthetic cortisol steroids (hydrocortisone), other cases result in further suppression of the adrenal glands by the treatment. In some cases this may be due to the dose not being monitored closely or not being dosed correctly (incorrect dose amounts). It is of most importance that this type treatment is administered by a qualified medical professional, who is knowledgeable in adrenal hormone replacement therapies. The physician would also need to be skilled in monitoring a patient's hormone levels while they are
 being treated. A patient considering the treatment should also be thoroughly informed about the possible risks and side effects.

Hydrocortisone Therapy in CFS Patients with low Cortisol Levels

In the year 1996, the U.S. National Institutes of Health (NIH) – Centers for Disease Control, conducted studies of Chronic Fatigue Syndrome patients, treating them with doses of hydrocortisone (synthetic cortisol) to replace sub-clinically low cortisol levels. The trial of cortisol replacement therapy followed other studies that found low cortsol levels in CFS patients compared to healthy controls (non-CFS participants). The study was an attempt to see if the cortisol supplementation would relieve CFS symptoms.

Over-replacing Cortisol can Cause the Adrenal Glands to Shut-down

The NIH study of cortisol supplementation in CFS patients concluded that in some of the participants, the drug significantly relieved their symptoms but an adverse effect of "adrenal suppression" (further decrease in adrenal cortical output) was seen in some of them after several weeks on the drug.

This resulted in the conclusion that cortisol supplementation was not a safe treatment due to the risk of the treatment causing significant adrenal insufficiency. The outcome of the trial may have been more favorable if lower doses had been administered because CFS patients have mild adrenal insufficiency and do not require full cortisol replacement as do those with full-blown adrenal insufficiency.

Testing Cortisol Levels

With the potential risks involved in cortisol supplementation, which includes increased risk for hypertension and elevated glucose levels (high blood sugar), Adrenal Fatigue patients should consider natural methods for increasing cortisol levels safely. There are a number of potential causes for sub-clinically low adrenal function, including CFS, as addressed in the previous subheading, chronic and inflammatory diseases, traumatic stress and emotional disorders. These conditions can however first result in increased cortisol levels before causing a significant drop in them.

These facts point to the importance in first testing to determine the cortisol level before assuming it to be low and in need of being increased. If borderline low or sub-clinically low levels are not found, then boosting cortisol levels might not be what is needed. If however test results reveal the need for adrenal support, adrenal supplements may provide the needed answer. If supplements are taken to improve adrenal function, it is also important to retest adrenal hormone levels at regular intervals to monitor the treatment.

Natural Methods for Increasing Cortisol Levels

Taking safe over-the-counter supplements that help strengthen fatigued adrenal glands is recommended as a first line of treatment, rather than resorting to cortisol steroids that pose potential risks. Supplements that specifically help boost the adrenals in producing more cortisol, would be "glycyrrhizic acid" which is found in licorice root extract products and "adrenal glandular" which is found in products processed from the adrenal glands of animals.

Most adrenal glandular products are hormone free however one brand available called "Isocort" contains trace amounts of cortisol in the pellets that are processed from the adrenal glands of New Zealand sheep. It is recommended that any supplement always be taken at the manufacturer's recommended-dose and that any supplement is approved by a physician who knows a patient's medical background.

CHAPTER 9:

Effective Adrenal Fatigue Treatments

Boosting Fatigued Adrenal Glands

Adrenal Fatigue is a stress-syndrome, meaning the adrenal glands become blunted or diminished in their ability to moderate stress but there are treatments that can help.

Adrenal Fatigue, the sub-clinical form of adrenal insufficiency is not at the level of severity that full blown adrenal insufficiency is but the symptoms can still seriously affect those who develop the condition. Following below, are therapies that have been found to be effective in treating Adrenal Fatigue, the sub-clinical type of hypoadrenia.

Proper Rest Promotes Healthy Adrenal Function

People suffering Adrenal Fatigue are typically those who push themselves too hard. They maintain schedules that overextend their energy levels.

When you combine this type of daily pace with not taking time for getting plenty of rest and proper sleep, Adrenal Fatigue can become a chronic issue. Symptoms of overextended adrenals can be improved and in some cases completely relieved by taking rest periods of a few minutes, at different points during the day. Labor laws in some areas of the world for example, require that employees are given breaks to rest and recharge their energy levels, at a rate of about 15 minutes per four hour shifts. Leisure and vacation time away from work duties is also an important aspect of getting proper rest.

Adequate Sleep can Boost the Adrenals

Getting proper sleep is also very important because studies have shown that during sleep the body repairs itself and replenishes hormone reserves that are responsible for all bodily functions and energy levels. The adrenal stress-hormone called "cortisol" is one of those hormones that requires proper sleep to maintain an adequate level of reserves for steady release throughout active daytime hours (circadian rhythm).

Studies have also shown that the body requires 8 hours of uninterrupted sleep per 24 hour cycle. Sleep that is fragmented (interrupted) may rob the body of the deep-stages of sleep the body requires.

Reducing Stress Increases Adrenal Hormone Reserves

Chronic stress is the strongest contributing factor in the development of Adrenal Fatigue. The adrenal glands moderate stress, by releasing cortisol which helps the body cope with and recover from daily stressors. When stressors are overwhelming, traumatic or chronic, this causes hyperactive use of cortisol which over time causes reserves of the hormone to diminish due to inability of the adrenal glands to keep up with the excessive demand. For this reason, reducing stress levels in every way possible is essential in successfully treating Adrenal Fatigue. Learning relaxation techniques, exercise routines, deep-breathing and stress reduction methods can be greatly beneficial in this area.

Eliminating Stimulants can Reduce Adrenal Stress

It is also important to remove stimulants from the diet whenever possible. Both caffeine and chocolate for example, can provide boosts in energy but afterward, an adverse drop in energy can occur. The same is true of other stimulants, including consuming moderate to large amounts of refined sugar and drinking alcohol. If stimulants are not limited or eliminated, Adrenal Fatigue sufferers may find that they experience ongoing dependency on them and a vicious cycle of highs and lows in their energy levels. It may become increasingly difficult for them to start their day without a stimulant, such as a cup of caffeinated coffee.

Adrenal Friendly Diet

A diet rich in healthy foods, including fruits, vegetables, nuts and grains (complex carbohydrates) can contribute to improved adrenal function and overall better health.

Eliminating foods containing refined sugars can also be beneficial because these types of "simple carbohydrates" supply quick-energy but afterward cause a crash and a feeling of being stressed-out as addressed earlier. Foods to avoid would be those that are manufactured and that contain refined sugars such as soft drinks, pies, cookies, cakes and candies.

Adrenal Boosting Supplements

Adding helpful over-the-counter supplements that contain adrenal-boosting properties, at the manufacturer's recommended dose can also help restore proper adrenal function. These would include vitamins B-5, B-5 and B12, with vitamin C also added which helps the B-vitamins absorb and work better in the body. Other natural supplements that have been found to help boost adrenal function and energy levels include herbals such as licorice root extract, ashwagandha, Co-Q10 enzyme, Asian Ginseng and Rhodiola Root. Beef (bovine) "adrenal glandular" which is usually hormone-free, comes from the adrenal glands of cows and processed into pill form and has also been reported to be effective in treating adrenal fatigue.

Talk to your Doctor

It is important to fully inform your doctor about any supplements you may choose to take, so that he can determine whether or not they are safe in adding them to any treatments you are currently undergoing. Monitoring for any unpleasant or concerning side effects is also important when adding a supplement of any kind to your treatment regimen.

CHAPTER 10:

Diagnosing and Treating Addison's Disease

Symptoms of Autoimmune Adrenalitis

While there are other types of adrenal insufficiency that fall under the category of "Addison's disease", the most common type is autoimmune adrenalitis. This type of adrenal dysfunction is full-blown, rather than mild as is experienced with Adrenal Fatigue. It is important that people, who believe they are experiencing true adrenal hypo-function rather than a milder form of Adrenal Fatigue, are properly tested by medical lab analysis.

Addison's disease is most commonly an autoimmune disorder affecting the adrenal glands. Each person has two adrenal glands, which are part of the endocrine system (hormone producing) and they sit on top of each kidney in a person's body. These glands are small and shaped like pyramids about the size of a walnut, measuring about 3 x 5 x 1 cm in size.

The immune system can mistakenly recognized these glands as intruders and begin to attack them (autoimmune response), slowly destroying them with auto-antibodies (killer cells from the immune system). This is the most common cause of Addison's disease.

Addison's Disease Results in Hormone Deficiency

When the onset of Addison's disease occurs, this causes the adrenal glands to become inadequate in supplying the important adrenal hormones needed by the body, the two major hormones being "cortisol" and "DHEA" (dehydroepiandrosterone). Symptoms of Addison's disease appear once at least 90% of the adrenal cortex (the protective outer layer of the gland) has been destroyed by the autoimmune process known as "autoimmune adrenalitis".

Addison's Disease Symptoms

The symptoms of Addison's disease are those of adrenal hormone deficiency. Addison's disease causes adrenal insufficiency, meaning a reduction in adrenal hormone production and output.

The Everything Adrenal Fatigue Book

As previously stated, the two major hormones that become low due to this disease process are cortisol and DHEA.

Cortisol is the "stress hormone" and "anti-inflammatory hormone" that gives the body its ability to handle and recover from stressors and inflammation. DHEA is a "sex hormone precursor", meaning the hormone that converts into testosterone, estrogen and other male and female sex hormones needed by the body.

When the adrenal hormones become low, a person may experience the following symptoms of low adrenal function.

• fatigue
• joint/muscle pain
• weight loss
• diminished appetite
• low blood pressure (hypotension)
• hyper-pigmentation (darkening of the skin)

If left untreated, people with Addison's disease are at risk of experiencing an adrenal crisis, meaning they can potentially go into shock and possibly coma or death.

The Everything Adrenal Fatigue Book

Diagnosing Addison's Disease

Addison's disease is most often diagnosed through blood testing and MRI (magnetic resonance imaging). Medical blood lab testing can measure the adrenal hormone levels and if they are found to be low, this can indicate adrenal insufficiency due to Addison's disease.

Patients will then usually be tested for adrenal function via an ACTH Stimulation Test. This test uses the ACTH hormone, which usually comes naturally from a person's own pituitary gland, to stimulate adrenal-cortisol hormone production but, during the test, it is administered to the patient by injection.

A patient will have a baseline blood draw taken before the test. After the ACTH hormone injection, they will have two or more additional blood draws taken at 30 minute intervals, and these three blood levels will then be compared. If the two or more additional blood levels of cortisol do not significantly increase above the baseline level, a diagnosis of adrenal insufficiency is confirmed.

Other tests that may be ordered would include an MRI to detect the extent of adrenal gland destruction, and a blood test to detect antibodies that the immune system is directing against the adrenal glands.

Treatment for Addison's Disease

Addison's disease is treated by replacing the low adrenal hormone levels. Once blood tests reveal which adrenal hormones are low, hormone replacement therapy will begin. One of the major hormones called cortisol, which is most commonly low in adrenal insufficiency states, must be replaced with a steroid cortisol substitute called a "corticosteroid" also referred to as "hydrocortisone". Patients will need replacement with this synthetic hormone and any others found to be low, for the rest of their lives.

Addison's disease patients are also usually required to wear a medical ID bracelet, so that if they experience an adrenal crisis (sudden, severe drop in adrenal hormones), the person finding them will know that they are treated for Addison's disease and that, they may need to have an emergency-dose of corticosteroid steroid administered by a doctor.

The Everything Adrenal Fatigue Book

There are a number of other causes of adrenal insufficiency, but Addison's disease is the most common, affecting about 1 in 100,000 people according to medical sources.

Anyone who suspects they may be experiencing symptoms of adrenal insufficiency should see their doctor for immediate evaluation.

CHAPTER 11:

How to Set Reasonable Health Goals

Resolving to Become Healthier

Most everyone has resolved at different times in their lives to live healthier through improved diet and exercise. Improving one's overall fitness is a wise resolution and is especially important for those who suffer health problems such as CFS, Fbromyalgia and/or Adrenal Fatigue.

Goals for becoming healthier are better achieved if they are reasonably set, with expectations being attainable rather than a near-impossibility to reach. Gradual improvements in diet, exercise and stress-reduction are those that are more easily attained and that are more successfully held onto and improved upon. Methods for pacing one's self to accomplish health resolutions at a successful pace will be addressed in the subheadings that follow.

Common Health Resolutions

Goals for better health are often referred to as "resolutions" and many people set them within days or weeks before the change of a new year. The following are goals that people making resolutions commonly desire improvement-in, for overall better health.

• weight loss
• a healthier, low-fat diet
• exercising to tone the body and improve stamina
• a plan for dealing-with and reducing stress

Many people have found through trial and error, that setting reasonable goals rather than ones that are very difficult to achieve, helps one to remain inspired to achieve them, rather than becoming discouraged before reasonable gains are made.

Improved Diet and Weight Loss

When improving one's diet for weight loss, the goal should also include the improvement of health. This would mean to not only eat less but to eat healthier foods as well.

Starvation diets, for example, are not healthy and can result in a person binge-eating once they see weight loss resulting and they are tempted to compromise their diet. Gradual weight loss has been shown in studies to be healthier and weight that is more easily kept-off, rather than regained.

Cutting out fattening foods by what is sometimes called the "cold turkey" method, in which they are stopped suddenly and completely may also be less successful for some dieters than a more gradual cutting-out of fatty foods. If a person resolves to completely remove white and sweet breads from their diet, for example, they might better achieve this by eating 50% less white bread at first and then cutting it back another 25% over a few weeks time and weaning off the last 25% within a few more weeks.

Unhealthy foods should also be replaced with healthy ones, to include vegetables, fruits, nuts and grains.

Reasonable Exercise Routines

Exercise is quite possibly the single healthiest pursuit one can undertake. Studies have shown that it not only improves muscular tone in the body and cardiovascular health but it can also improve one's emotions and help to reduce stress levels.

Whether one begins an aerobics or calisthenics exercise regimen, they should do so at a pace their bodies can tolerate well. Extending beyond one's tolerance level can result in bodily injury and unnecessary fatigue. By beginning a low-impact and safe level of exercise, one can gradually build the level as they are able to safely adjust to it. Walking is a safe way to begin a cardiovascular, aerobics exercise routine, building speed and distance at a gradual pace. Low repetition calisthenics, using no weights, then slowly graduating to light weights and heavier weights can be a safe method for a body toning routine.

Reducing Stress

No one is immune to the effects of stress in everyday life but it can be reduced and maintained at a healthier level through stress-reduction practices. This area of improvement for better health takes time and effort to achieve but can contribute both to improved physical and emotional well-being.

As mentioned in the previous subheading, exercise is a great natural stress-reducer. Other methods for reducing and gaining control over stress include enjoyable pastimes and hobbies such as art pursuits and leisure activities. The following are hobbies and leisure activities that can be enjoyed while reducing stress levels.

- writing
- painting
- sculpting
- hiking
- camping
- games
- music
- reading

Taking time out to simply rest quietly or to meditate can also contribute to stress reduction. These activities can have a cumulative effect toward conquering stressors that exert negative effects on mental and physical health.

In conclusion, it is wise when making resolutions for better health, to include all three areas of improvement as addressed in the previous subheadings. Each of these can contribute to the success of the others for a well-balanced improvement in overall health.

CHAPTER 12:

When is DHEA Supplementation Beneficial?

The Non-prescription Adrenal Hormone Treatment

With some adrenal insufficient states, it is the DHEA hormone that is deficient but under what conditions is it safe to replace the low hormone via supplementation?

DHEA is an essential adrenal hormone that carries out a number of important purposes in the body. The hormone can become low due to certain types of disease processes, such as autoimmune, inflammatory and chronic health disorders but also decreases in the body with age. Levels of DHEA can drop below normal values or remain in a low-normal state, which may require hormone replacement therapy. When DHEA is supplemented when it is not needed, it can cause adverse effects in the body.

What is DHEA?

The full medical name for this hormone is "dehydroepiandrosterone" and is a hormone that is endogenous, meaning it is made in the human body, even though it can be supplied to the body from an outside source. Being the most abundant adrenal hormone in the body, it is manufactured by the adrenal glands and afterward is converted into other essential hormones, as they are needed. It is also referred to as a steroid but because it undergoes a synthesizing process in the brain, it is also called a neurosteroid.

DHEA is available over-the-counter in supplement form and most brands are made from extracts derived from wild Mexican yams. Claims by some medical sources and by research done by firms that manufacture DHEA supplements, the hormone can increase positive mood, sex drive, immune system function and energy levels when supplemented. It is important to add that these benefits would only be realized if supplementation with the hormone is done so at the dose needed and at a level that does not adversely affect sex hormone balance.

Precurser to Sex Hormones

A major function of DHEA is converting into sex
hormones for both males and females. All sex
hormones are common to both sexes but in
different balance for each gender. The male
hormones DHEA converts into are referred to as
androgens and the female hormones it converts
into are referred to as estrogens. Because of the
hormone being available to convert into these
other hormones this also places it in the category
of being a "precursor hormone", meaning it is on
stand-by to convert as needed.

Hyperandrogenism in Men and Women

It is important that DHEA levels are in proper
balance in women, due to the risk of too many
male hormones being produced through
conversion if levels become too high. The term
for too much male hormone production is
"hyperandrogenism" and can result in a condition
called hirsutism in women, in which there is
excessive growth of body hair.

Other symptoms of hyperandrogenism in women can include acne, increased muscle growth, a change in sex drive, decreased breast size and a deeper tone to the voice. Some medical sources state that about 10% of the female population is experiencing some degree of hirsutism from hyperandrogenism.

A major cause of hyperandrogenism in women is "polycystic ovary syndrome" (PECOS) in which the ovaries cause an excessive amount of androgens to be produced. It can also be caused by overproduction of DHEA from the adrenal glands, from over-supplementing with DHEA or from taking doses of the hormone when it is not needed.

Hyperandrogenism can also occur in males but symptoms and manifestations of the condition are less noticeable in adult males. When symptoms do occur, they can include male pattern baldness (alopecia), acne, abnormally high testosterone levels, changes in sex drive and irritability. In pre-teen males, hyperandrogenism can cause early onset and an abnormal increase in the advancement of puberty.

Testing Before Supplementing

With the risk of inducing hyperandrogenism from supplementing with DHEA when there is not a need for it, this points to the great importance in first testing the hormone's level before attempting to increase it in the body. Adrenal hormone testing usually includes both the DHEA and cortisol levels because these hormones interact with each other, creating a ratio between them. According to some medical sources, DHEA can suppress cortisol levels and vise-versa and supplementing one may also require supplementing the other to keep the ratio balanced.

Opinions vary as to what a safe supplemented amount of DHEA would be. Some sources state that up to 25mg in females and up to 50mg in males is a safe dose however, this would not be the case if DHEA levels are already at proper-normal, high-normal or flagged-high.

Supplementation added at these levels, could cause adverse side effects as previously described and demonstrates the importance in testing adrenal and sex hormone levels before considering supplementation.

The Everything Adrenal Fatigue Book

A patient can test hormone levels and supplement with DHEA on his own if levels are low but should do so with extreme caution, making sure to retest the hormone levels at regular intervals to monitor the treatment. The better and safer scenario would be to have a treating doctor order saliva and/or blood-serum adrenal and sex hormone tests, to assure that DHEA supplementation is safe for a patient and so that he can determine the proper dosage needed.

SECTION THREE – (Pages 120 – 177):
"Natural and Prescribed Treatments for Adrenal
Fatigue"

CHAPTER 1:

Adrenal Fatigue by Any Other Name

Many Doctors pronounce patients "normal" in
regard to their adrenal function when they pass
the tests they feel are the only ones needed to
diagnose low adrenal function. These will often
be the "ACTH Stimulation test" and/or a snapshot
blood cortisol reading (the major adrenal stress
hormone). The problem is that adrenal fatigue is a
condition of disrupted "cortisol rhythm" and is not
necessarily due to cortisol being low all of the
time or because the adrenals can't be stimulated.
Adrenal fatigue is not usually found until a multi-
reading test is performed to gauge a patient's
readings of cortisol, over a 24 hour period. Even a
test that takes two readings - one at morning upon
waking when cortisol levels are supposed to be
highest and one at midnight when levels are
supposed to be lowest can help to give a cortisol
average, rather than just a single snapshot level.

What really convinced me years ago, that mild adrenal dysfunction does exist and has been proven in medical research, are those medical research articles published in regard to syndromes like CFS (Chronic Fatigue Syndrome), Fibromyalgia and PTSD (Post Traumatic Stress disorder). These articles clearly state that people with these type syndromes often suffer low cortisol levels and they have also found strong association of these syndromes to chronic stress, of either the prolonged type or the type caused by sudden traumatic events.

Here are example research article quotes:

"Several years ago, Dr. Straus and his colleagues found that CFS patients had slightly lower levels of circulating cortisol, the major glucose-regulating stress hormone, than did healthy individuals. Doctors have long believed that even subtle deficiencies in cortisol can result in lethargy and fatigue." (http://www.niaid.nih.gov/news/newsreleases/1998/pages/cfs.aspx)

"Both fibromyalgia and CFS are often viewed as being stress-response related, and abnormalities of the HPA axis have been found in both disorders.

...

In our study, morning cortisol levels were lower in women with CFS than in healthy controls. Some studies of the HPA axis in CFS show a mild hypocortisolism of central origin, in contrast to hypercortisolism of major depression.

...

Cortisol levels peak in early morning and need to be collected before patients rise in the morning; and determining single levels of hormones that are secreted in a pulsatile fashion may not be representative of normal functioning." (http://www.medscape.com/ -- "Cortisol and Hypothalamic-Pituitary-Gonadal Axis Hormones" © 2004 BioMed Central, Ltd. verbatim copying and redistribution permitted)

"Post-traumatic stress disorder is often associated with low production of cortisol." (http://psychiatry.jwatch.org/cgi/content/full/2007 /1210/1)

While research articles do not use the term "adrenal fatigue", this is exactly what is being described by them. They will instead use terms such as "mild adrenal insufficiency", "blunted HPA axis", "hypocortisolism" or simply "low cortisol".

These type research articles are out there in significant numbers, so doctors who still do not believe that sub-clinical adrenal insufficiency conditions exists, need to take a look at a few of these published studies.

Adrenal fatigue by whatever other name they wish to call it does exist and is found in a variety of stress-related syndromes.

CHAPTER 2:

Adrenal Fatigue and Thyroid Patients

A lot of patients with thyroid disease also have some co-existing adrenal fatigue.

Add to thyroid disease, something like a traumatic or very stressful even and you can really suffer from adrenal fatigue. Your circadian rhythms are off with this condition and are why sleep patterns may also become disrupted. Your cortisol and DHEA (the two major adrenal hormones) will have their peaks, at the wrong times, such as at sleep time and your normal drop in these hormones also happens at the wrong time, like during the day, when you most need the peak-energy. Adrenal fatigue that continues for a long period of time (chronic) may then become "adrenal exhaustion" and this is the point to where you no longer experience those needed peak levels at all.

I have had adrenal fatigue for several years, as a feature of Chronic Fatigue Syndrome and co morbid to my autoimmune thyroid disease (Hashimoto's thyroiditis) and I have also experienced adrenal exhaustion. Mine turned into adrenal exhaustion, after experiencing the onset of hypothyroidism and at the same time, I had gone through a period of severe, prolonged stress.

Mine did not improve when I first began thyroid hormone replacement but actually worsened for a time. After several months on the correct thyroid dose, I finally saw some improvement in thyroid and adrenal symptoms. At times of extra stress and extended periods of hard physical activity, I've taken some adrenal support supplements, that I learned about when researching about adrenal fatigue and these have helped a great deal. These include multi "B" vitamins, especially B-12, in sublingual form (liquid) and vitamin C, magnesium, selenium, zinc, DHEA 25mg (over-the-counter adrenal hormone) and sometimes but less often, an Adrenal Cortex Extract (processed beef adrenal glands in pill form).

These always help me greatly during flares of adrenal fatigue but I don't take the ones containing actual trace amounts of adrenal hormone (cortisol), as a permanent regimen. However, as safe as they are supposed to be at the recommended doses, it likely would not hurt for me to do so if I felt it was necessary at some point.

I considered taking a cortisol drug called "Cortef" (natural adrenal steroid) and had a Dr. willing to treat me with it but I was slightly wary of steroids, even at low doses and I still am. I have however, read many reputable medical resources that state that Cortef is safe as physiological doses (25mg and less), to supplement a person's low cortisol levels from adrenal exhaustion but the hormone drug can cause "adrenal suppression", if administered in full replacement doses (above 25mg but may vary) and if used for extended periods of time. In my opinion, adrenal support supplements are safer and usually all that is needed for most cases of adrenal fatigue.

How does a patient know if they have adrenal fatigue? Blood adrenal hormone levels can be helpful but are like a "snapshot reading" as mentioned previously and since cortisol levels go up when you are stressed, such as at a blood draw, this can affect the snapshot blood level.

This is one of many reasons why saliva testing is recommended because you can conveniently obtain several cortisol-level readings over a 24 hour period to establish the adrenal hormone rhythms.

Saliva testing has been researched and found very accurate by reputable medical groups; in fact it is used to monitor hormone levels in medical research, including that done by World Health Organizations. It is also an approved form of testing, by many major health insurance companies, such as Blue Cross/Blue Shield.

Many pharmacies carry the type manufactured by "ZRT Labs, Inc.", which is also an approved blood lab, so you might check with your pharmacy to see if they carry this brand. Most adrenal saliva tests are not terribly expensive and can be diagnostic in detecting adrenal fatigue.

CHAPTER 3:

Balancing Adrenal Fatigue Treatment with Hypothyroid Therapy

Adrenal Fatigue can be a real dilemma for thyroid patients in many ways and my belief is that this is why some doctors like to stay away from it and one of the ways they do this is by denying its existence.

Medical sources including the thyroid medication manufacturers warn that "untreated adrenal cortical insufficiency" (low cortisol) can be worsened by treating hypothyroidism with hormone replacement therapy, without first correcting it or treating them both simultaneously. What then becomes a question is - how bad does the low cortisol have to be, to present a real problem? Certainly full blown adrenal insufficiency can present this problem but it only takes common sense to realize that severe adrenal fatigue or adrenal exhaustion can as well (low cortisol regardless of cause).

Less severe adrenal fatigue many times will resolve when hypothyroidism is corrected because the low functioning thyroid causes everything, including the adrenal glands to operate low in the body (slowed metabolism). When adrenal fatigue in hypothyroid patients isn't severe, it usually corrects on its own when the hypothyroidism is corrected.

Other patients aren't as fortunate and you can find their testimonials often online. They struggled with their adrenal fatigue worsening when they started thyroid hormone medication and continue to struggle with it as they continue their treatment. Some of them also have intermittent adrenal fatigue that is ingoing or chronic and flares easily with stress or physical exertion, even while they are on optimal thyroid hormone therapy. I personally fit into that category and I had a variety of symptoms that worsened with the start of thyroid hormone medication. I feel it's possible that many of the patients, who report worsening symptoms for a while after starting thyroid medication for hypothyroidism, may very well be experiencing these adjustment symptoms as both the thyroid and adrenal hormones are trying to correct to normal levels.

The Everything Adrenal Fatigue Book

Those who seem to never reach a well adjusted state on thyroid hormone should have their adrenal hormones tested in my opinion.

In regard to cortisol steroids (corticosteroids) that replace low cortisol which include the brands "Prednisone" and "Cortef". I agree with those sources that warn if a doctor is not highly skilled in administering these drugs for adrenal fatigue, they can potentially worsen it (adrenal suppression). I am not adding this fact as anti-cortisol treatment propaganda. I am mentioning it because this warning is a logical one in regard to the administering of steroid treatments of any kind! True adrenal insufficiency is easier to treat in one sense because patients need full replacement as a lifelong treatment, while adrenal fatigue sufferers need less than full replacement and usually for short term. It's possible there is a dose of cortical steroid that is safe to treat adrenal fatigue on a permanent basis but medical research has yet to find it, so that it works for a large cross section of people, safely and with no adverse effects or risks.

If safe over-the-counter supplements can be tried first, this is a better way to treat adrenal fatigue in my opinion. A doctor will be needed for corticosteroid treatment as previously mentioned, if it also needs to be administered for severe adrenal fatigue cases at a certain point. Helpful over-the-counter supplements for adrenal fatigue include the "B" vitamins, especially B-5, B-6 and B-12, vitamin C, licorice root extract (only as label-recommended) and processed adrenal glandular supplements (usually beef/bovine source), using the same precautions as with licorice root.

Some people report improvement while on herbal adrenal support supplements as well, including use of a supplement called "Adreset", made by the Metagenics Company. This company also makes a vitamin supplement for adrenal support called "Cortico-B5 & B6", which also contains magnesium and vitamin C in it. My pharmacist, who works with local doctors, recommended these to me because they are pharmaceutical grade and they have helped with my flares of adrenal fatigue a great deal.

A company that makes a non-hormone adrenal glandular is Vitamin Research Product Company who offers their product called "CortiTrophin". Their company has Pharmacists and MDs behind research and development of their supplements and is why I believe they are more reputable than some of the other adrenal supplement manufacturers that out there.

Much of the medical community still has this condition on a back shelf, until it becomes more widely accepted as a real illness.

CHAPTER 4:

Adrenal Fatigue or "Hypocortisolemia"

With Adrenal Fatigue being one of my areas of interest, I watch for updated research in regard to this subject. Many times I will come across medical research articles in regard to this syndrome but it will be referred to by other names, such as "mild adrenal insufficiency" or simply a "low cortisol state". Some reputable medical entities still do not believe that an Adrenal Fatigue type disorder exists (less that full-blown adrenal insufficiency), including surprisingly, the Mayo Clinic (a source I highly respect).

With Adrenal Fatigue, as with more severe adrenal adrenal insufficient states, the hormone "Cortisol" is most commonly the one that becomes low or deficient. It is the hormone that manages stress in the body on a daily basis and provides energy for the body, in a cyclic rhythm. In the recent medical research article I will refer to below, it is referred to as "hypocortisolemia" (low cortisol).

It seems as if some in the medical community avoid the term "Adrenal Fatigue", for reasons I have yet to understand. I do believe in the case of some medical people, they feel anything less than true, full-blown adrenal insufficiency, simply does not exist and so anything recognized that is less than this more severe form of adrenal dysfunction, is a pseudo-syndrome (not legitimate) in their opinion. The problem I have with this attitude is the fact that a number of research articles going back more than two decades, recognize mild adrenal dysfunction or sub-clinically low functioning of the adrenal glands. This includes research articles on Chronic Fatigue Syndrome (CFS), Fibromyalgia and Post Traumatic Stress Disorder (PTSD), which have all been proven in a number of medical research studies, to present with low cortisol levels.

There have in fact been trials of treatments for these disorders, using a cortisol replacement drug (hydrocortisone), with some results being favorable and some that were not favorable, which could be a matter of finding the correct therapeutic dose of the drug, that will relieve symptoms without adverse side effects.

In studies of PTSD patients, there have been favorable outcomes using cortisol replacement in controlled studies, to manage the symptoms of this stress disorder. The research article I refer to below, also points this out.

I do not believe it is a coincidence that these syndromes that present with low cortisol, including; CFS and PTSD, are also referred to as "stress syndromes". I also believe that Adrenal Fatigue is a low-cortisol, stress-syndrome and strongly associated with these other syndromes.

The medical research article I wish to refer to is titled; "Stress-induced hypocortisolemia diagnosed as psychiatric disorders responsive to hydrocortisone replacement" (U.S./NIH - PubMed Website).

It is an interesting medical research article in that, it points out the fact that severe early life stressors, can result in later life cortisol hormone deficiencies that are mild-to-moderate. The article also points out that this mild adrenal insufficient state they refer-to in the article as; "hypocortisolemia", is often mistaken for psychiatric disorders.

The Everything Adrenal Fatigue Book

This correlates with the fact that many people who suffer Adrenal Fatigue, attest to the fact that their symptoms were considered to be psychosomatic, before they were thoroughly tested for cortisol levels and found to be deficient.

This research article recommends testing hormone levels, including cortisol, before prescribing psychotropic medications (antidepressants). A major importance of the article as well, is the fact that low cortisol that is not severe enough to be true adrenal insufficiency, is again recognized. Some of us choose to call this sub-clinical hypo-functioning of the adrenal glands; "Adrenal Fatigue". If medical professionals prefer a different term then they should officially name the syndrome, so that more people in the medical community will recognize it, test for it and treat it.

CHAPTER 5:

CFS, Fibromyalgia and Low Cortisol

For more than two decades, researchers studying Chronic Fatigue Syndrome (CFS) and Fibromyalgia Syndrome, have conducted studies in regard to adrenal function in patients with these syndromes and have concluded that patients are found to be experiencing "low adrenal function" as one of the features of these syndromes. This co-existing condition is also called "adrenal fatigue", "adrenal exhaustion" and "low adrenal reserve". Reputable medical sources also state that patients with Thyroid Disease are at higher risk than the general population, for also having co-existing CFS and/or Fibromyalgia.

Through testing of a patient's adrenal hormones, it can be determined if that person has low-functioning adrenals. In addition to blood testing, saliva tests are also accurate for testing the "free levels" of the adrenal hormones, the main ones being DHEA and cortisol. A "24 hour urinary cortisol test" can also be done to test adrenal-cortisol levels.

Another major adrenal function blood test is also available, called the "ACTH Stimulation Test". This one is designed to confirm or rule out true "adrenal insufficiency" (full blown). Most CFS and Fibromyalgia patients do not have true, full blown adrenal insufficiency but a milder form of adrenal fatigue/exhaustion.

Conclusions by major medical research groups, including the NIH, state that low cortical levels, are found to be a contributing factor in CFS/FMS, due to dysfunction of the HPA Axis (Hypothalamus-Pituitary-Adrenal Axis). It is my opinion because of this, that CFS/FMS has as one of its features, a form of adrenal fatigue, that does not meet the definition for true "adrenal insufficiency" and because of this, it cannot be medically treated the same. With full blown Adrenal Insufficiency, the low adrenal hormones must be replaced through steroid treatment (cortisone-steroid/hydrocortisone). With lesser forms of low adrenal function, such as adrenal fatigue, steroid treatment can possibly worsen the adrenal problem because the steroids may cause "adrenal suppression".

This means the patient may have to take the steroids, the rest of their life because anything less than very short-term use of the steroids, can cause this suppression.

This milder form of low adrenal function, many times is treated with supplements such as DHEA, adrenal glandular and multi-vitamins that contain those that help boost adrenal function, as well as B-12 shots. These are all over-the-counter supplements, with the exception of B-12 shots but you can also obtain B-12 in oral form that is over-the-counter. All of these supplements have been found to be helpful in resolving adrenal fatigue conditions.

Some of the other things medical researchers have studied in regard to CFS and Fibromyalgia, is the fact that these syndromes can have different triggers for different patients but with many, it is an underlying viral, autoimmune, bacterial etc…, type infection in the body, that causes chronic activation of the immune system and over time, this uses up some of the adrenal reserves.

The adrenals serve a major role in releasing cortisol, the body's natural anti-inflammatory, attempting to ward off inflammation. Cortisol (also called "cortical"), is also the "stress hormone", that helps the body to deal with stress of all kinds, without it, even the smallest stressor would cause shock and death (adrenal crises). It, along with adrenaline, are "fight or flight" hormones and help protect the body from the effects of stress, from minor emotional stress, to major ones, such as a car accident or a serious disease.

This in my opinion is why persons with CFS/FMS have such low tolerance for stressors both emotional and physical. With low adrenal function, even mild emotional and physical stressors result in major fatigue. Couple this with the immune system dysfunction that CFS/FMS patients also experience and you have syndromes with serious symptoms that can greatly impact quality-of-life. It may be that the immune deficiency found in both CFS and Fibromyalgia is also a type of burn-out of that system, due to constant, ongoing activation of it, that the body eventually loses the ability to continue.

The Everything Adrenal Fatigue Book

As with all other opinions about CFS and Fibromyalgia, we have to consider all of the above, as some of the many theories that are out there however, I feel the evidence of low adrenal function in CFS and Fibromyalgia, is overwhelming. What I have described, is what I feel connects these syndromes to a form of adrenal fatigue.

CHAPTER 6:

Conditions That Cause Mild Adrenal Insufficiency

Adrenal insufficiency is a condition in which the adrenal glands do not produce enough hormones to aid in regulating the body's metabolism, stress coping, controlling inflammation and sexual functioning. The main adrenal hormone that becomes low with this condition is "cortisol," as mentioned in previous chapters and when low levels are detected in a person, it is sometimes referred to as "hypocortisolemia". Full blown adrenal insufficiency is referred to as "Addison's Disease." There are, however, milder forms of adrenal dysfunction as listed below. Some statistics state that about 10% of people with thyroid disease experience a degree of mild adrenal insufficiency.

Post Traumatic Stress Disorder. This condition, abbreviated PTSD, is a traumatic stress-caused condition that is also considered to be an anxiety disorder.

People experience the onset of this disorder as a result of severe traumatizing experiences, such as car accidents, acts of violence that are perpetrated upon them, the sudden loss of a loved one or having been in active combat during wartime. The severe shock caused to the body from such incidents can cause the glands regulating adrenal hormone output to become "blunted", meaning they begin to function at a sub-normal level. While their adrenal hormones may remain within normal limits, they will be at lower or lowest normal (borderline low), which causes them to have an inability to cope with stressors.

Research studies on PTSD that are published by reputable medical groups (including the U.S. National Institutes of Health) state that low cortisol levels found in patients with this disorder contributes to their symptoms of anxiety, insomnia and flashbacks, meaning they may mentally relive their traumatic experiences repeatedly. In controlled test studies, using cortisol supplementation to treat PTSD patients, results showed that symptoms were reduced significantly by carefully monitored physiological dosing to increase their low level of the stress hormone.

Chronic Fatigue Syndrome (CFS). This condition has also been found to cause a low level of the stress hormone cortisol evidenced by analyzing the blood and urine cortisol levels in people who experience the illness. Research studies on CFS have repeatedly confirmed this fact and have also found that patients report that they were experiencing chronic or sudden severe stress just before the onset of the illness. This would mean that CFS is very possibly also a stress-related condition that causes the adrenal hormone regulating glands in the body to become blunted.

The U.S. National Institutes of Health released a report in October of 1996, in which they found through a controlled study, that cortisol supplementation/replacement in patients with CFS had a benefit but was found to be short-lived. Afterward, some patients began experiencing a more severe form of adrenal suppression, meaning it caused a worsening of their adrenal insufficiency after a few weeks on the cortisol replacement drug.

Fibromyalga Syndrome (FMS). Being very similar to CFS, Fibromyalgia also has fatigue as a major symptom. The aspect that sets this illness apart from CFS is the widespread body pain that is not found to be as prominent in CFS patients. Despite this fact, researchers studying both illnesses have found them to have 75% crossover similarities. This includes the fact that FMS patients often report chronic stress as being a factor in their development of the illness.

A number of research studies have also found cortisol levels to be low in FMS patients and controlled trials of cortisol supplementation have been conducted to determine if there would be a benefit for these patients. The findings were similar to those found when supplementing CFS patients with cortisol hormone replacement and while some patients improved, the long-term risks for using the drug did not merit establishing it as a medically recognized treatment for FMS.

Adrenal Fatigue. This sub-clinical form of adrenal insufficiency is still not recognized widely by the medical community, although certain types of doctors recognize the disorder.

This includes MDs who practice holistic treatments, Naturopaths and Osteopathic Physicians. With this syndrome which is also referred to as a condition of "low adrenal reserves" and "adrenal exhaustion", many of the symptoms found in CFS and FMS are not present, including joint and muscle pain and other inflammatory problems in the body. Adrenal Fatigue is strictly a condition causing mild to moderate fatigue and reduced stress tolerance. Some medical sources are stating that adrenal fatigue that is prolonged and not treated, through proper rest, improved diet, adrenal boosting natural supplements and reducing contributing stressors, may result in the condition becoming a precursor (a pre-condition) to CFS and FMS.

While the conditions listed above are commonly found to cause mild adrenal insufficiency, other conditions can also be a cause or contributing factor, including other chronic, inflammatory and autoimmune diseases that contribute to increased stress levels in the body. See a professional, licensed physician for a complete evaluation if you suspect that you may be suffering from a health condition causing mild adrenal insufficiency.

CHAPTER 7:

Cortisol & DHEA Supplements for Adrenal Fatigue

Since the year 2004, I have written a lot on the subject of mild hypo-cortisolism that is found in different conditions, that for lack of another well-established term, we call "adrenal fatigue" but it is often during the research I'm doing at any given time for articles etc..., that I often find, that many in the medical community, still do not recognize mild forms of adrenal insufficiency and they do not believe that adrenal fatigue syndromes exist.

I actually hope Doctors or medically knowledgeable people of any type, will at some point make a suggestion for a name that doesn't come across as bogus for the syndrome and at the same time, if they don't believe sub-clinical forms of adrenal hypo-cortisolism exist, to also explain why all of the research articles that describe it, are somehow all collectively wrong on the subject (the later challenge will be much more difficult).

The majority of adrenal fatigue patients will at times have snap-shot readings that are normal, when blood tested for cortisol levels and they will also pass the ACTH Stimulation Test (confirms or rules out full blown adrenal insufficiency) and is why it is recommended to obtain multiple readings throughout the day, via saliva cortisol testing for milder forms of adrenal hypo-cortisolism.

When I personally had the ACTH Stimulation Test performed on me, my cortisol reading was about mid-range on the baseline reading however, I was anxious before and during the test and it's better to obtain cortisol rhythm of multi-readings during a normal activity day. Even though I had a normal baseline on that ACTH Stimulation Test, I also had a 24 hour urinary test through an Endocrinologist's Office and my cortisol averaged "10.7", with normal range at the lab being <119 for males ages 18 and above. To be in the middle of that range (mid-level), I would have had to have a result of about a 50 or 60 and my Dr. admitted that mine was a very low reading for a 24 hour urine cortisol test.

This confirmed that I didn't have true, full-blown adrenal insufficiency but that I did have a serious case of adrenal fatigue.

In medical research studies, in which patients with different diseases, are found to have low cortisol levels, the medical investigators are usually referring to "low cortisol" as being in the low-normal range, so is low compared to "controls" and low compared to normal subjects. They even give the number differences, calling them "significant" even when the difference is only 2 or 3 points lower than normal subjects have.

One statement the NIH makes in their Centers For Disease Control study of CFS, that has always struck me as important is this one; "Doctors have long known that even subtle deficiencies in cortisol is associated with lethargy and fatigue" (Oct, 1996).

How Does DHEA Supplementation Factor into This?

I've lately come more to the conclusion that I've suspected from the beginning of my search and research on adrenal fatigue, that supplementing with DHEA, will help low DHEA levels but usually doesn't help with low cortisol. Maybe in some patients it does help to raise cortisol, once the circle of conversion goes completely around but there's conflicting info about DHEA out there. What will help the adrenals to produce more cortisol, are vitamins that support adrenal function, rest and adequate sleep and if needed, the safe and cautious use of licorice extract and adrenal glandular extracts. Some Doctors also sometimes prescribe; pregnenolone to adrenal fatigue patients or other combinations of hormones.

A lot of medical resources state that the majority of women can safely take 25mg or less of DHEA and there is very low risk of it causing their androgen levels (male hormones) to go too high and men are supposed to be able to take up to 50mg safely.

I don't feel DHEA would suppress cortisol to a significant degree at these doses but the point is that they also might not help raise cortisol, so that taking it alone, could cause more of a DHEA to cortisol ratio imbalance. This isn't true of people who have low DHEA but normal cortisol levels because DHEA is all they need in these cases. The Journal of Pharmacology has a research article that states that patients with Crohn's Disease and Lupus, are one example of low DHEA, that when supplemented, improves symptoms of these diseases but DHEA can become low for other reasons as well.

In Some Cases Cortisol Supplementation is the Answer

The "American Psychiatric Association", made a statement in the "American Journal of Phychiatry", in a research test that was conducted by 3 psychiatrists and 6 MDs. They stated that supplementing Post Traumatic Stress Disorder patients (PTSD) with low-dose cortisol, can help them because they found that the low cortisol, is a major factor in causing symptoms of the illness.

This study, which didn't go overboard with the dosing of cortisol, like other studies have in the past, such as those experimenting with cortisol supplementing in CFS patients, had more favorable results at the lower-dose treatment.

There are now newer studies reported by the major medical research publishing groups that show that CFS patients did improve with lower-dose cortisol treatment. These studies are more recent than those that reported "adrenal suppression" and other adverse effects at higher dose treatments.

Cortisol replacement therapy is only available by prescription, by a licensed medical professional but hopefully as more research is done, they will find a safe dose that will help treat adrenal fatigue type syndromes.

CHAPTER 8:

The Role Stress in Diseases and Syndromes

Stress is a known trigger for adrenal fatigue and related syndromes, such as Chronic Fatigue Syndrome and Fibromyalgia and can also bring an autoimmune disease to the surface that is in the body but hasn't fully manifested. Thyroid diseases are some of the more common health disorders that can be triggered by stress, especially Grave's Disease/hyperthyroidism.

PTSD (Post Traumatic stress Disorder) is also a chronic stress caused syndrome and is also classified as an anxiety disorder.

I personally went through an extreme period of chronic stress and my thyroid disease, called "Hashimoto's Thyroiditis", manifested as a result as well as a severe case of adrenal fatigue. I was left untreated for these disorders for several months and as a result experienced a severe flare-up in the year 2003 that also triggered the onset of Chronic Fatigue Syndrome.

I initially developed a severe case of hives and a strange viral type illness that left me with the co-occurring CFS. Afterward, the lymph nodes in my neck remained mildly swollen to this day and I also suffer multiple chemical sensitivities (MCS).

My belief is that CFS is a syndrome causing an altered HPA Axis (Hypothalamus-Pituitary-Adrenal glands), plus altered immune system function (deficiency). I suggest to people who suspect they have adrenal fatigue, CFS or a chronic illness/disease to have their adrenal hormones and all other hormones (including the sex ones) checked as well because it is my belief that hormonal imbalances over time, can possibly result in CFS and Fibromyalgia type illnesses.

Some who have read my articles online or my posts on forums, may wonder why I have the passion I do for the adrenal syndrome subjects and it is because it is my belief that adrenal fatigue can eventually cause CFS and/or FMS type syndromes, when not diagnosed and treated early when diagnosed.

Another strong association to these type syndromes is EBV (Epstein-Barr Virus), which causes mononucleosis initially in some patients but afterward, remains in a persons body for life. This virus is suspected of having a strong connection to CFS. While most people have EBV in their system beginning in childhood (estimates are 80 to 95% of the population), most only have antibody titers to the virus, that are just barely positive, like a "5", a "10", "20" above normal, etc..., others actually have flare-ups of this virus (reactivation), probably due to a compromised immune system (immune deficiency) that causes high titers of the virus to replicate in their bodies over time.

Many in the medical field are of the opinion that EBV is a background virus like many others in the herpes virus-family that can flare repeatedly like cold sores can (also a herpes virus that remains in the system). When flare-ups happen, they believe it can cause or at least contribute to symptoms of CFS in some people.

In my case, my EBV antibodies count was "218" with normal range being <20, so mine was more than ten times the normal cut off range.

Some Doctors believe the EBV test means nothing, unless actually being used to test for mononucleosis but there has to be a reason some patient's EBV counts elevate so highly. Both MDs who treat me for hypothyroidism and CFS, believe that EBV can flare/reactivate in some patients who have the higher titers of the virus in their system. Many sources also state that adrenal fatigue is a major feature of this because the adrenal glands are the major moderators of the immune system.

While EBV may not be the actual root cause of CFS, it has been shown to be an indicator of immune dysfunction in studies that have been conducted. In my opinion, it is just one of many factors that can contribute to the symptoms of CFS.

The Centers for Disease Control/U.S. Gov., has been publishing studies and diagnostic criteria for CFS, for many years, so it is recognized as a real illness.

Many patients with CFS have complete remission of it within two to five years while others have partial but significant improvement, even if it never completely remits. Some may have it for many years but regardless, it does not cause organ damage or decrease life span expectancy, according to published medical research. It also does not negatively affect intellect; despite the "brain fog" symptoms it also causes in patients who experience it (i.e. difficulty concentrating and short term memory loss).

Things that speed recovery for CFS, are; treating the associated adrenal fatigue, getting proper sleep and rest, a healthy diet, exercising to tolerance and making sure other diseases a patient might have are treated. Under-treatment of a thyroid disorder for example, can serve as a trigger for continuing CFS flare-ups and may actually be a trigger for the syndrome itself according to some medical sources. Many sources also state that thyroid patients commonly have co-occurring CFS and/or Fibromyalgia (CFS & FMS have 75% crossover symptoms).

CHAPTER 9:

Another Look at Adrenal Fatigue Treatments

There are non-steroidal treatments that can help resolve adrenal fatigue as previously mentioned, including supplements, such as an over-the-counter adrenal hormone called "DHEA", which when taken at the recommended dose, will convert into other needed hormones, including the sex ones. I will add that with DHEA, you need your doctor to help you decide what dose-level is safe for you via testing of your current blood level of the hormone.

There are also "adrenal glandular extracts" that contain animal adrenal glands, usually bovine (beef) that have been reported for many years to help patients regain normal adrenal function. There is also "licorice root extract", that research has found helps patients with adrenal fatigue, to produce higher levels of the stress regulating hormone; "cortisol". An important energy-producing enzyme called "Co-Q10" can also be a beneficial supplement.

Multi-vitamins and minerals can also be very helpful, especially the "B' vitamins (like B-12, B-5 & B-6) and minerals such as magnesium, potassium, and zinc.

Why in the world these things that might be called "natural remedies", are sometimes given a "bad rap", I'll never know! I feel it is ludicrous for anyone, including someone who is a medical professional, to feel something must be a synthetic in order to be effective. This is an incredible view since the vast majority of what keeps us healthy, are nutrients that occur naturally. Let's give God or Nature (if you prefer), the credit for having enough sense to provide us with a few things to keep us healthy and to heal us!

I am not against synthetic medications, they are lifesavers and tremendously effective but when the idea is implied that there is no treatment for a condition, unless it is severe enough to be treated with a synthetic, I will disagree 100%. It is sometimes claimed that pharmaceuticals are the only available treatments and there are obviously other helpful non-prescription treatments available.

The Everything Adrenal Fatigue Book

It is a complete and total shame, to allow patients who can benefit from these, to continue suffering rather than giving them a trial of them.

Natural versus Pharmaceutical? – Both should be Options

I'll just make a few more statements, hopefully that point to the fact that there are no perfect answers for many aspects of this debate in regard to "natural versus pharmaceutical" although there is a general guidance we all know to follow that even common sense points out to us.

Licensed medical practitioners obviously are those called to heal and treat people who have illnesses and to keep them well (preventative). The first line of reasoning is to see a doctor when you need medical treatment. Conventional medicine and pharmaceutical drugs have saved lives, extended lives and restored quality of life.

Natural remedies have had miraculously positive and healing effects on some people as well, that conventional treatments failed to resolve.

Some natural supplements are far safer than others and just as with pharmaceuticals, they do not have the same effect on each individual. Some people have been known to have severely adverse effects from naturals and others have died from them.

The same is true of some pharmaceuticals. SSRI antidepressant labels for example are now required by the FDA to include mention that some people have become suicidal when taking the drugs, especially younger people. I know for a fact cases of suicide have occurred in those prescribed the drugs but is rare. Does this mean SSRI's should be sloughed-off as harmful? Absolutely not, - some people could not survive without them.

On the other hand, naturals cannot be sloughed-off either and in fact, they were placed here by God or nature if you prefer for the very purpose of healing and keeping things well. Pharmaceutical drug-evolution actually came from natural remedies in many cases.

Now, in regard to articles and e-books (like this one) on the subject of health treatments, both natural and prescribed; there are simply too many "ins and outs" for any one side of the argument to claim they have the best answers on all aspects. That's almost like saying there is only one correct or perfect political or religious view on all aspects of those controversial subjects. It is simply not going to happen.

Even in the medical field, certain types of MDs do not see Osteopath doctors as being as legitimate as other types of MDs and others do not recognize naturopaths as being legitimate at all. This despite the fact that they can be legally accredited after required studies to practice with a license in those fields. As far as "quacks" go, and I say this respectfully, there are quacks in every field, including MDs, Natural Remedy people, police officers, ministers, dentists, article/e-book writers, etc...

Never should this fact cause us to see everyone in light of the bad apples that exist in their fields. Moderation should be done, in all of these fields.

The Everything Adrenal Fatigue Book

MDs have to answer to medical boards, ministers to the clergy of their denomination and article writers, to the websites they write for.

What's my point? Well, I first of all feel it doesn't hurt to have these type discussions in-balance for perspective-sake. I do believe however that there are and never will be perfect answers for every aspect of this subject. I wish there were always definitive answers but this is simply not true in many cases. That's life and the world we live in and also why we have to maintain our individuality and make thoughtful decisions the best we can and then pray (or hope) for the best outcome.

My Own Positive Experiences with Natural Supplements

I have mentioned previously, my positive experiences with supplements that help significantly when I experience flares of adrenal fatigue. I have seen benefits with naturals among my family members as well.

My wife suffered severe yeast infections for 15 years that were intermittent but caused lots of agony when they did occur. She went to several doctors and each recommended prescriptions, some that helped temporarily. One of the last doctors she went-to prescribed a dangerously long regimen of Diflucan (ten 200mg pills taken for 10 days). The reason she did not have the prescription filled is because the pharmacist's jaw almost fell to the ground when he saw the prescription and told her if she took the highest dose for 10 days, irreversible liver and/or kidney damage could potentially occur.

Someone had been recommending she take probiotics and acidophilus (natural supplements) and she finally took the advice and upon taking a regimen of these two natural supplements had complete recovery from the yeast infections. She was absolutely thrilled.

Even this example is not to say every person would see the same results but made us realized naturals cannot be dismissed.

Some things in the natural category are absolutely needed, which includes Vitamin B12 that if some people did not take, would cause them to die from pernicious anemia. The same is true with people who need iron for other types of anemia and calcium supplementation due to parathyroid imbalance etc...

Pharmaceuticals can have the same life-saving, sustaining and healing benefits so I feel doctors should be willing to see a balance between the two in cases when either or both can benefit.

Determining when, a conventional treatment is better than a natural treatment and vise versa, can be a difficult subject with lots of details and factors involved. Some issues involving the conventional Vs natural treatments debate include disagreements about when they should be combined or when one is a better option than the other, etc.... and really becomes complicated at times. Patients are often caught in the middle not knowing which direction to turn. Those suffering severe symptoms from health disorders and diseases as I also have at times are very willing to look at every possible legitimate avenue to find relief.

In short, there are not always simple answers although we all wish the way was unmistakably clear in every case.

One thing I have always made sure of is to mention in each article or e-book I've written that includes reference to natural supplements (non-prescription, over-the-counter), that patients run them past their doctors before taking them. I've always done this going back six years to my beginnings in writing on health subjects because I know that all treatments don't have the same effect on each and every person.

I mention in a recent article a test a person can do at home using one drop of iodine on the soft area of their arm and observing the spot it makes to see if the iodine absorbs quickly or slowly. When quickly absorbed, this possibly indicates the thyroid is starving for iodine or is in need of more due to inadequate thyroid hormone production. I gave a lot of thought into adding this self-test into the article I was writing because there are doctors out there who disagree that the iodine spot test has any legitimacy whatsoever.

I also mention several times in the article that tests like these cannot diagnose and that only qualified doctors can diagnose thyroid disorders.

The reason I added mention of this test into the article however was for several reasons, one of which I will now describe:

I called-in live, to a health T.V. show, on which Dr. Sherri Tenpenny was a guest, back in about the year 2003 or 2004 (still have the show on tape) and told her I had three abnormal readings on some thyroid lab tests, that were done due to symptoms of an under active thyroid I was having but that my doctor at the time was delaying treatment because my TSH was not reaching "10.0 or higher" (pituitary hormone that elevates with hypothyroidism). It in fact it was at "8.3" (my T3 uptake was also flagged low) but she mentioned that if my case was caused by Hashimoto's thyroiditis, there could also be antibodies blocking thyroid hormones. She suggested I do an in-home iodine spot test using Lugol's solution (iodine product).

I bought a bottle of the iodine and had my non-thyroid diseased family members to also place iodine drops on their inside upper arm areas at the same time I did. Their spots stayed for an entire day, while mine absorbed within one-hour. I waited a few days and did the test again with same results (very fast absorption). I then had blood testing for thyroid antibodies a few months later (immune cells that cause disease) and Hashimoto's thyroiditis was revealed, my anti-TG ABs coming in at "537" with normal range being "<35". Both my TPO and TG ABs are highly elevated when re-rested each year but I am at least now treated for my thyroid disorder. I was amazed that Dr. Tenpenny accurately predicted my case as being autoimmune thyroiditis.

Dr. Tenpenny is Board Certified in emergency medicine and is an osteopath doctor and very well-known and recognized as an expert in many areas, including vaccinations. These type MDs can not only be board certified but can perform surgeries, deliver babies etc... .

I found however that some MDs in other fields look at osteopaths almost in the same category as naturopaths when they are in-fact qualified in far more areas of practice. My point being that there are qualified doctors in both the conventional and natural medical fields and many practice aspects of both.

CHAPTER 10:

The Importance in Confirming Treatment Information

Some non-pro medical subject authors (like me) do a good job in relating information about available treatments because they have thoroughly researched. I also agree that articles on medical subjects should be backed by information that can be confirmed but for perspective and balance on this issue and by no means wanting to come across offensive, let me add the following.

One of the major reasons non medical professionals have resorted to search, research and writing medical-subject articles, is due to their not being reasonably informed about their medical conditions by their doctors. Doctors are overbooked and overworked and they simply do not have the time to educate patients beyond the very basic things. Some readers at this point of this chapter might ask "Why would a patient need to know details of their health disorders anyway?" The answer is, first of all because they have a right to know.

The illnesses they experience in many cases are life-altering, possibly debilitating and lifelong. Secondly, doctors can give incorrect diagnoses and whether everyone who may consider this aspect wants to believe it or not, patients many times find corrected diagnoses because they become self-educated enough to spot a wrong diagnosis.

Giving myself for example, I am an autoimmune thyroid disease patient who was diagnosed with hypothyroidism in 2003 but first experienced a period of hyperthyroidism. The first two doctors I went to, resorted to snap diagnoses and prescribed antidepressants, claiming my problems were emotional. Strangely, many of my symptoms didn't match those of anxiety and/or depression even though I stated them clearly (i.e. very dry skin, sudden rapid weight loss with no change in diet, hair breaking off, muscle weakness etc…….). I finally literally had to demand blood testing and the thyroid disease was revealed immediately, including highly elevated auto-antibody levels.

After diagnosis, I was under-treated for two years
by doctors who did not know how to properly
administer thyroid hormone replacement therapy.
How do I know this? Because an Endocrinologist
I finally made an appointment with was appalled
at the bad treatment I was receiving, once
reviewing my medical records. These type things
are why I began search and research extensively.
Let me add that I've had doctors tell me I was
incorrect about something I researched on very
reputable medical sources and upon inquiring
with other doctors, found that the initial doctor
was incorrect on some very important things.

In regard to my health articles, I can say with
absoluteness that anything found in them can be
confirmed. I in fact will not include anything in
one that can't be confirmed by numerous
reputable, reliable sources (medical ones). On
very rare occasions I will mention speculation and
will state it as such, also mentioning that medical
research has yet to find the definitive answer.

Just to add one more example in this area, I'll refer to another thyroid patient advocate and fellow adrenal fatigue sufferer named Mary Shomon, who is also not a medical professional but a very professional writer of medical subjects. Her story is very similar to mine, in that she was forced to research due to difficulty getting doctors to order proper blood testing and afterward difficulty in receiving proper treatment. Since my own self-educating, I have corresponded with 1,000s of patients (not an exaggeration) and have heard my story reflected back to me in their similar experiences. Most were offered antidepressants as I was before diagnostic testing revealed what treatment was actually needed. They would not have even known what to ask for had they not become proactive and self-educated.

I realize I did not start this part of the chapter talking about medical doctors per se but about medical writers, however, most write for the benefit of other medical professionals. It is almost as if patients are not given the benefit of the doubt for having some intelligence of their own and as if some medical people literally try to withhold information from patients.

They are in-essence saying "Put your complete trust in us and don't ask questions and don't double check us (confirm)." If some patients did not do this however, they would not have received treatments that sometimes were lifesaving. This is not meant as disrespect but there are medical practitioners who fall short. This is why people resort to second opinions. There are also fantastic doctors out there (the majority) but without at least some education on the part of patients, they might not know whether a doctor is good or is one who is about to let them go down hill very fast health-wise.

By no-means was this meant to degrade the medical profession (Thank God for them!) but I felt it very important to explain why in my case, I began to share needed info with fellow-patients. Money had absolutely nothing to do with it and I wrote online for two years not seeking compensation of any kind. I had and do have genuine compassion for others who are going through what I went through before being properly treated for thyroid disease and adrenal fatigue.

I believe health articles written by non-medical professionals should be confirmed within reason, as long as motives for doing so are always genuine and not an attempt toward censorship. The vast majority of online medical-subject articles are by non-medical professionals as it is and I'm sure there are unreliable ones out there. I also believe there are some medical ones, written by professionals that contain unreliable information as well. Some of the medical fields have strong disagreements with each other as well, such as conventional MDs who do not agree with holistic approaches used by some Osteopath doctors, etc...

You can see from this and other of my articles that this is an area of heart for me. The bottom line is that some patients are in desperate need of information and sometimes need to hear from fellow-patients they can relate-to.

Finally in closing this e-book - my suggestion to thyroid patients, who begin thyroid hormone replacement medication and have a negative reaction to it, is to ask for tests of their adrenal hormone levels.

Not only can your Doctor order blood tests of your adrenal hormone levels but there are also home "saliva tests", that are available via, online mail order and through Pharmacies that medical research has concluded are as accurate for testing the "free levels" of circulating adrenal hormones as serum blood tests are. One company that offers adrenal saliva test kits online and through many pharmacies nationwide is "ZRT Labs, Inc." founded by biochemist and breast cancer researcher, David T. Zava, (PhD).

Confirming the existence of adrenal fatigue is the first important step toward getting proper treatment for symptoms and to possibly see complete recovery from this common but serious stress related syndrome.

(END)

www.ingramcontent.com/pod-product-compliance
Lightning Source LLC
Chambersburg PA
CBHW020421290526
45785CB00002B/668